AFTER 40, YOUR BODY IS NOT BROKEN

A Structure-First Reset for Posture, Mobility, Strength, and Pain-Free Training

ADRIAN WELLS

Founder, DominionBuilt

Built on Structure. Refined Through Precision.

DominionBuilt Press

Published by DominionBuilt Press
First Edition
ISBN 979-8-9962455-2-9
dominionbuilt.co

CONTENTS

Introduction

Your Body Is Not the Enemy

There comes a point after 40 when your body can start to feel different.

Not always all at once.

Sometimes it happens slowly.

You wake up and feel stiffer than you used to. You stand up from a chair and notice your hips do not open the same way. Your shoulders feel tight. Your back feels guarded. Your knees talk more than they used to. One side feels stronger than the other. A workout that used to make you feel alive now leaves you feeling beat up for days.

And somewhere in the back of your mind, a question starts forming:

Is my body breaking down?

That question can feel heavy.

Because it does not only sound physical. It can feel personal.

You may start wondering if you waited too long. If you missed your window. If getting older means you have to accept stiffness, weakness, pain, and decline as the new normal.

But before you accept that story, you need to hear this clearly:

Your body is not the enemy.

What feels like failure may actually be feedback.

What feels like weakness may be a signal.

What feels like stiffness may be your body protecting areas that no longer move, stabilize, or carry load the way they should.

And what feels like "getting old" may sometimes be the result of years of compensation building quietly underneath the surface.

Age is real.

Recovery changes. Muscle changes. Joint tolerance changes. Energy changes. Your body may need more wisdom, more preparation, and more intentional training than it did when you were younger.

But age is not the whole story.

Many people over 40 are not simply dealing with age. They are dealing with structure.

They are dealing with posture that has shifted over time. Mobility they slowly stopped using. Weak links their body has learned to work around. Training programs that ask for more output without ever checking the foundation underneath the movement.

Then one day the body says: I cannot keep compensating like this.

That is when things start to feel confusing.

You stretch, but the tightness comes back. You train harder, but the pain moves somewhere else. You rest, but the stiffness returns. You try a new workout, but it feels like your body cannot find the right muscles. You do what worked for someone else, but your body does not respond the same way.

That can make you feel broken.

But often, the issue is not that your body is beyond repair. The issue is that you have been trying to solve a structure problem with random effort. And effort without structure can become frustration.

The Problem With Most Fitness Advice After 40

Most fitness advice starts in the wrong place.

It starts with intensity.

More reps. More sweat. More discipline. More motivation. More workouts. More pushing.

But after 40, more is not always better. Sometimes more just exposes what has been ignored.

More squats will not fix poor hip control. More stretching will not fix poor stability. More core exercises will not fix a ribcage and pelvis that cannot organize together. More shoulder work will not fix an upper back that barely moves. More cardio will not fix a body that feels unstable under load.

This is why so many adults over 40 feel trapped. They are not unwilling. They are not lazy. They are often doing more than people realize. But they are doing it without a clear map.

They are told to stretch what feels tight, strengthen what feels weak, and push through what feels hard. But the body does not work in isolated pieces. The body works as a system.

Your neck can be affected by your upper back. Your low back can be affected by your hips. Your knees can be affected by your feet. Your shoulders can be affected by your ribcage. Your strength can be affected by your posture. Your mobility can be affected by your stability. Your pain can be affected by compensation.

That is why a structure-first approach matters.

What Structure-First Means

Structure-first means you stop asking only:

"What exercise should I do?"

And you start asking:

What is my body showing me?

It means before you chase a harder workout, you look at the foundation underneath the workout.

How do you stand? How do you breathe? How do your shoulders sit? How does your spine move? Can your hips open? Can your feet create stable contact with the floor? Can your body control its own range of motion? Can you move without borrowing from the wrong places?

Structure-first does not mean you avoid strength. It means you earn better strength. It means you do not build on compensation and call it progress.

At DominionBuilt, the principle is simple:

Structure governs strength.

Strength is not only about how much weight you can lift. Strength is also about whether your body is in a position to produce force safely and consistently.

A body with poor structure can still be strong. For a while. But eventually, compensation collects a cost. That cost may show up as tightness, irritation, weakness, asymmetry, poor recovery, or a feeling that your body is always one wrong movement away from flaring up.

A structure-first reset does not promise perfection. It gives you a better starting point. It helps you see the difference between a body that is broken and a body that has been compensating.

That distinction matters. Because if you believe your body is broken, you may give up. But if you understand your body has patterns, you can begin to address them.

The Map This Book Gives You

This book is not here to shame you. It is not here to tell you that everything you have done is wrong. It is not here to turn your body into a medical project. It is here to give you a clearer map.

That map starts with three areas:

Upper Chain. Core Stack. Base.

Your head, neck, shoulders, ribs, pelvis, hips, knees, and feet are not separate problems. They are connected parts of one system. When one area loses position, mobility, or control, another area often compensates.

This book will help you see that chain more clearly.

You will learn why your body may feel different after 40. You will learn how posture, mobility, stability, and strength connect. You will learn why stiffness can be information. You will learn why pain should not be ignored or blindly pushed through. You will learn how the upper body, core stack, and lower body influence each other. You will learn why assessment matters before programming. You will learn simple reset routines you can begin using. You will learn how to build strength without breaking yourself down.

And most importantly, you will learn how to stop guessing.

This book will not diagnose you. It will not replace a doctor, physical therapist, or qualified professional when you need one. But it will help you think more clearly about your body. It will help you ask better questions.

Who This Book Is For

This book is for the adult over 40 who feels older than they should.

It is for the person who used to move better and wants to know what changed.

It is for the person who feels stiff every morning, whose shoulders round forward, whose hips feel locked, or whose back tightens during workouts.

It is for the person who wants to get stronger but does not want to keep getting hurt.

It is for the person who has tried programs that worked for other people but did not fit their body.

It is for the person who knows they need to move, but no longer trusts their body the way they used to.

This book is not for people looking for shortcuts. It is not for people who want hype. It is not for people who want to punish their body into submission.

It is for people who want to rebuild with wisdom.

How To Use This Book

Read this book as a map. Do not rush through it looking for the perfect exercise. The exercise is not the whole answer. The understanding matters.

The first part of this book will help you understand why your body may feel different and why structure comes before strength. The second part will help you read the body in sections: the upper chain, the core stack, and the base. The third part will help you reset posture, mobility, and control.

As you read, pay attention to the sections called "What This Explains." Those sections are designed to help you connect what you feel in your body to structural patterns that may be contributing to it.

Again, this is not diagnosis. It is direction. The goal is not to label yourself. The goal is to understand what may be happening so you can stop guessing.

The First Shift

Before we go further, make one shift.

Stop seeing your body as the problem.

Start seeing your body as a messenger.

A tight muscle may be telling you something. A weak pattern may be telling you something. A painful movement may be telling you something. A repeated limitation may be telling you something.

Your body has been keeping records. It has been adapting to how you sit, stand, breathe, train, recover, carry stress, avoid movement, and compensate around old patterns.

Now you are going to learn how to listen differently.

Not with fear. Not with frustration. Not with shame.

With structure.

Before you can rebuild, you need to understand why your body started feeling different in the first place.

And that begins with a simple truth:

Your body is not broken.

It needs a better map.

Part One

Understanding Your Body

CHAPTER 1

Why Your Body Feels Older Than It Should

Here is what that looks like in practice. A person in their mid-40s comes in after years of consistent training. They are not sedentary. They have not stopped caring. But the squat that used to feel natural now requires a warm-up that takes longer than the session used to. The shoulder that was never an issue now talks during pressing. The low back that recovered in a day now takes three. Nothing broke. The body just became less tolerant of the same inputs that used to be fine. That is not failure. That is information.

There is a difference between getting older and feeling older than you should.

Getting older is real.

Your body changes with time. Recovery may take longer. Muscle does not stay as easily as it once did. Joints may need more preparation. Sleep, stress, nutrition, workload, and training history all start to matter more than they did when you were younger.

That part is normal.

But feeling stiff every morning, guarded every time you train, uneven from side to side, or nervous that one wrong move will flare something up is not something you should automatically accept as "just age."

Aging may be part of the picture.

But it may not be the whole picture.

Many adults over 40 feel older than they should because their body has been adapting for years without being properly assessed, reset, or rebuilt.

The body adapts to what you repeatedly do.

It adapts to how you sit. How you stand. How you sleep. How you train. How you recover. How you compensate around old injuries. How you avoid movements that no longer feel safe.

Over time, those adaptations shape the way you stand, move, recover, and train.

Posture affects mobility. Mobility affects stability. Stability affects how much strength your body can safely express.

When that chain is ignored, the body often finds another way to get the job done.

And not every workaround is harmless forever.

Sometimes what feels like decline is really compensation that has been allowed to run too long.

The Body Keeps Adapting

Your body is always learning.

It learns from repetition.

If you sit for years with your head forward and your shoulders rounded, your body learns that position.

If you avoid deep hip movement for years, your hips learn a smaller range.

If one side has been carrying more load because of an old injury, your body learns that pattern.

If your breathing becomes shallow because of stress, tension, or poor posture, your ribcage and trunk can learn to stay guarded.

The body is not passive. It is always adjusting.

The problem is that every adjustment has a cost.

At first, compensation can be helpful. If your ankle is stiff, your hip or knee may help you get through the movement. If your upper back does not rotate well, your low back may borrow extra motion. If one glute does not contribute well, your hamstring or low back may help finish the job. If your core does not stabilize well, your body may create tension somewhere else to feel safe.

That is your body trying to protect you.

But protection can become limitation.

A compensation that helps you get through one season can become the reason your body feels restricted in the next one.

This is why so many people feel confused after 40.

They are not always dealing with one dramatic injury. They are dealing with years of small adjustments. A little less mobility here. A little more tension there. A little less strength on one side. A little more guarding in the low back. A little more stiffness in the morning. A little more hesitation before certain movements.

Over time, those small changes start to add up.

Then the body feels older than it should.

Stiffness Is a Signal

Most people treat stiffness like an enemy. They feel tight, so they stretch. Sometimes that helps.

But when the same stiffness keeps coming back, the body is usually asking for a closer look.

Stiffness may mean a joint is not moving well. It may mean a muscle is protecting an unstable area. It may mean your body does not trust a certain range of motion. It may mean one area is working too hard because another area is not doing its job. It may mean your posture, breathing, or movement patterns are creating constant tension.

This is why random stretching often fails.

If tightness is only a flexibility problem, stretching may help. But if tightness is a protection strategy, stretching alone will not solve the root issue.

The body may tighten again because it still does not feel supported.

For example, tight hip flexors may not only mean your hip flexors need stretching. They may also connect to pelvic position, poor glute control, weak trunk stability, sitting habits, or the way you stand and walk.

Tight traps may not only mean your traps need massage. They may connect to forward head posture, poor rib position, shallow breathing, weak upper-back control, or shoulders that do not sit well on the ribcage.

Low-back tightness may not only mean your back is the problem. It may connect to poor hip mobility, poor bracing, weak glutes, limited upper-back movement, or a body that has learned to protect itself with tension.

This does not mean every tight muscle has a hidden cause. Sometimes you are simply stiff.

But when stiffness becomes repeated, stubborn, or connected to movement problems, it deserves attention.

Do not ignore it. Do not panic over it. Read it with more clarity.

Weakness Is a Signal

Weakness can also tell a story.

After 40, many people notice that certain muscles do not respond the way they used to. They train legs, but feel everything in their knees or low back. They do core exercises, but never feel their core working. They train shoulders, but their neck takes over. They do glute work, but feel hamstrings, hip flexors, or low back instead. They try to get stronger, but one side always feels different.

This can be frustrating.

But weakness is not always just lack of effort. Sometimes weakness is poor access.

Your body may not be able to use a muscle well because the position around it is poor. A muscle can only work as well as the structure allows.

If your ribcage and pelvis are not stacked well, core and glute connection can change. If your shoulder blade does not move well, pressing and pulling can feel off. If your foot cannot create stable contact with the floor, your hip and knee mechanics may suffer. If your hips are restricted, your low back may work harder than it should.

This is why simply adding more exercises does not always fix the issue.

More glute exercises do not guarantee better glute function. More core exercises do not guarantee better trunk control. More shoulder exercises do not guarantee better shoulder mechanics.

The body needs the right position, the right control, and the right progression.

That is why weakness should not only be judged by how much weight you can lift. It should also be judged by whether your body can access the right muscles at the right time.

Pain Deserves Respect

Pain is more serious than stiffness or weakness. It should never be ignored. It should never be used as a badge of honor. And it should never be blindly pushed through.

Pain is a signal that deserves respect.

That does not mean pain always means damage. But it does mean your body is asking for wisdom.

One of the biggest mistakes adults over 40 make is waiting too long to listen. They feel a small warning, but keep pushing. They feel a repeated ache, but call it normal. They feel one side moving differently, but ignore it. They feel a sharp signal, but try to train around it without understanding it.

Then the body gets louder.

The goal of a structure-first approach is not to make you afraid of movement. The goal is to help you respond with wisdom.

Some discomfort during training can be normal. Effort is normal. Muscle fatigue is normal. Learning new movement can feel awkward.

But sharp pain, increasing pain, joint instability, numbness, tingling, swelling, or symptoms that do not settle should not be dismissed.

This book is not here to diagnose pain. But it is here to help you stop treating pain like an inconvenience with no meaning.

Your body speaks through signals. Pain is one of the signals that requires the most respect.

Why Old Workouts Stop Working

Many people over 40 try to return to the workouts that used to work. They go back to the same lifts. The same running plan. The same bootcamp intensity. The same body-part split. The same "push through it" mindset.

But the body they are bringing into those workouts is not the same body they had at 25 or 30.

That does not mean it is worse. It means it has history.

Training history. Injury history. Posture history. Stress history. Movement history. Recovery history.

And that history affects how it responds.

A workout that was productive years ago may now expose restriction, instability, or compensation.

Someone may return to squats thinking their legs are the issue, when the real limitation is hip control, ankle mobility, or a trunk that cannot brace well under load.

The exercise is not bad. The entry point is wrong.

This is why some people feel betrayed by their body.

They think: "I used to be able to do this."

That may be true. But the answer is not always to force your way back. The answer is to rebuild the path.

You may still be able to train hard. You may still be able to get strong. You may still be able to improve your body dramatically. But the starting point matters more now.

After 40, your body often demands a smarter entry point. Not because you are weak. Because you have less room for careless programming.

The Wrong Starting Point

When people feel their body slipping, they usually start in one of three places.

They stretch more. They train harder. Or they stop moving.

Each response makes sense. But each one can miss the real issue.

Stretching more can help if the problem is simple tightness. But if the stiffness is coming from poor control, poor positioning, or compensation, stretching may only give temporary relief.

Training harder can help if the problem is deconditioning. But if the body is moving through poor patterns, more intensity may make the compensation stronger.

Stopping movement can help if the body needs short-term rest. But if you stay inactive too long, the body may lose even more capacity, confidence, and range.

The better starting point is assessment.

Not medical diagnosis. Not overanalysis. Assessment.

Look at what your body is showing you. Where do you feel restricted? Where do you feel unstable? Where do you feel uneven? Where do you feel strong? Where do you lose control? Where does tension keep returning?

This is how you begin to stop guessing.

You do not need to know everything. You need to start paying attention to the right things.

WHAT THIS EXPLAINS

If your body feels older than it should, it may not be because everything is falling apart. It may be because your body has been compensating longer than you realized.

This may explain why stretching gives temporary relief but the tightness comes back. The issue may not only be the tight muscle. It may be the reason the muscle keeps tightening.

This may explain why workouts that used to help now leave you feeling beat up. Your body may be trying to perform without the same mobility, stability, or recovery it once had.

This may explain why one side always feels different. Your body may have built a pattern around an old injury, dominant side, posture habit, or weakness you never fully addressed.

This may explain why certain exercises never feel right. Your structure may not be giving you access to the position, control, or muscle connection the exercise requires.

This may explain why you feel stuck. You may not need more random effort. You may need a better map.

The First Reframe

The first step is not to panic.

The first step is to reframe what your body is showing you.

Stiffness, weakness, unevenness, fatigue, poor recovery, and pain are all signals worth reading with more clarity.

Your body is not just failing. It is communicating. The question is whether you know how to listen.

That is what this book is building toward.

Not fear. Not obsession. Not self-diagnosis.

Clarity.

Because before you rebuild strength, you need to understand what strength is built on.

That is where we go next:

Structure.

Your body may feel different after 40. But different does not mean broken. It means the map needs to change.

CHAPTER 2

Structure Governs Strength

Here is what structure governing strength looks like in a real session. Two people performing the same row exercise. One pulls correctly — drives the elbow back, keeps the neck out of it, and the shoulder blade moves cleanly. The other uses the same weight but the trap jumps first, the neck tenses, and the shoulder blade barely moves. The second person is working harder and getting less training effect — because the structure underneath the movement is borrowing from the wrong places. More weight will not fix that. Better structure will.

Strength is not just muscle.

That is one of the most important truths to understand after 40.

Most people think strength begins with effort. Lift more. Push harder. Add weight. Do more reps. Stay disciplined.

Effort matters.

But effort alone does not tell the whole story.

A person can work hard and still feel stuck. A person can train consistently and still feel beat up. A person can build muscle in one area while another area keeps tightening, aching, or compensating.

That is because strength does not happen in isolation. Strength is expressed through structure.

Your joints, posture, mobility, stability, breathing, alignment, control, and recovery all affect how much strength your body can produce and how well your body can tolerate that strength over time.

This is why two people can do the same exercise and have completely different outcomes.

One person does a squat and feels their legs, hips, and core working together. Another person does a squat and feels their knees, low back, and hip flexors take over. Same exercise. Different structure.

One person presses overhead and feels strong through the shoulders and upper back. Another person presses overhead and feels neck tension, low-back arching, and pinching in the shoulder. Same movement. Different foundation.

The exercise is not always the problem. The structure underneath the exercise may be the issue.

At DominionBuilt, the principle is simple:

Structure governs strength.

Before you ask your body to produce more force, you need to understand whether your body is positioned to handle it.

Why Strength Needs a Foundation

Strength is often treated like a numbers game. How much weight can you lift? How many reps can you do? How many days per week do you train? How hard did you push?

Those numbers matter. But they are not the whole foundation.

A stronger body is not only a body that can lift more. A stronger body is a body that can produce force with control, repeat the movement with consistency, recover from the work, and build capacity without constantly breaking down.

That requires structure.

Think of your body like a building. If the foundation is shifted, the walls may still stand for a while. The building may still function. But stress collects in the wrong places. Doors stop closing smoothly. Cracks show up. Weight is no longer carried evenly.

The building is not useless. It just needs the foundation addressed before more load is added.

Your body works in a similar way.

If your posture is poor, your joints may not line up well. If your mobility is limited, your body may borrow motion from another area. If your stability is weak, your muscles may guard instead of move freely. If your breathing is shallow, your trunk may stay tense. If your control is poor, your strength may leak.

Then when you add more intensity, the body does not simply get stronger. It may get better at compensating.

That is why a person can train for years and still feel like certain problems never change. They may be building strength on top of a structure that does not support the work.

Position Comes Before Power

Before your body produces force well, it needs position.

Position does not mean perfect posture. It does not mean standing stiff, pulling your shoulders back all day, or trying to hold your body in one ideal shape.

Position means your body has access to a more organized starting point.

Your ribcage and pelvis can work together. Your feet can connect to the ground. Your shoulders can move without your neck taking over. Your hips can move without your low back doing all the work. Your joints can stack well enough to transfer force.

When position is poor, the body can still move. But it may move with more effort than necessary.

For example, if your head sits forward and your upper back is stiff, your shoulders may not have the same freedom to move. Pressing, pulling, and reaching may start to involve more neck tension than they should.

If your ribcage flares and your pelvis tips forward, your low back may become the area that absorbs the stress during core work, squats, hinges, or overhead movements.

If your feet collapse inward and your hips do not control rotation well, your knees may take more stress during lunges, stairs, or running.

These are not moral failures. They are structural realities.

The body will use the position available. If that position is limited, unstable, or poorly controlled, the body will find another way. That is compensation. And compensation can make strength feel harder than it should.

Control Comes Before Load

Once position improves, control comes next.

Control is your ability to own a movement. Not rush through it. Not fall into it. Not bounce out of it. Own it.

Can you lower with control? Can you pause without losing position? Can you move through range without pain or panic? Can you keep breathing while the movement gets difficult? Can you feel the right muscles contributing? Can you repeat the same pattern again and again?

This matters because load reveals truth.

When you add weight to a movement, the weight does not only challenge your muscles. It challenges your structure.

If your body already moves with poor control, more load can expose the problem quickly. The knee caves in. The low back arches. The shoulder shrugs. The neck tightens. The hips shift. The feet lose pressure. The body finds the easiest way to complete the task.

You may not need more weight yet. You may need more control.

This is where many adults over 40 get into trouble. They remember what they used to lift. They remember what they used to tolerate. They remember how hard they used to train. So they return to the load before rebuilding the control.

But your body does not care what you used to do. It responds to what you are prepared for now.

That is not discouraging. It is clarifying. Because once you rebuild control, strength has a better place to go.

Mobility Gives Strength Access

Mobility is not separate from strength. Mobility gives strength access.

If you cannot access a position, you cannot build reliable strength there.

If your hips cannot move well, your squat, hinge, lunge, and gait will all be affected. If your upper back cannot extend or rotate well, your shoulders may not move well. If your ankles lack mobility, your knees and hips may have to compensate. If your ribcage and pelvis do not organize well, your core and glutes may not connect the way you expect.

This is why some people feel weak in positions they never train. The body does not feel safe there. It does not own the range. It does not trust the position. So it either avoids it, guards it, or borrows from somewhere else.

That is why stretching alone is not enough. Flexibility may help you access a range. But mobility is the ability to control that range. And strength is the ability to produce force inside that range.

Those three things are connected.

A structure-first body does not chase mobility for its own sake. It restores the range needed for better movement, better training, and better daily function.

You do not need to move like a gymnast. You need enough usable range to live, train, and build strength without constant compensation.

Stability Protects Strength

Stability is what allows strength to feel safe.

When the body does not feel stable, it creates tension. That tension may show up as tightness, guarding, or hesitation.

A joint that does not feel supported may not allow full power. A trunk that cannot stabilize may make the low back work too hard. A hip that cannot control motion may cause the knee or foot to compensate. A shoulder blade that does not move well may cause the neck to grip during upper-body training.

This is why stability matters. Not because you need to do fancy balance drills. But because your body needs to trust itself.

Stability gives your nervous system confidence. It tells the body: We can control this.

Without stability, intensity can feel threatening. With stability, strength has somewhere to land.

This is why a person can feel instantly stronger when their position and control improve. The muscle did not magically grow in one session. The body simply found a better way to organize force.

That is the power of structure.

Breathing Is Part of Structure

Breathing may not seem like strength work. But it matters.

Breathing affects rib position. Rib position affects trunk control. Trunk control affects pelvic position. Pelvic position affects hip function. Hip function affects lower-body strength.

The chain is connected.

If your breathing is shallow and your ribcage stays lifted, your body may live in a state of constant tension. That can make bracing harder. It can make core work feel disconnected. It can make the low back feel overused. It can make your body feel like it cannot relax or stabilize well.

Good breathing does not mean complicated breathing drills. It starts with awareness.

Can you breathe without lifting your shoulders every time? Can you exhale without collapsing? Can you feel your ribs move? Can you stack your ribcage and pelvis without holding your breath? Can you maintain position while breathing under effort?

This is not about becoming obsessed with breathing. It is about realizing that your structure includes more than muscles and joints. Your breath helps organize your body. And a better-organized body usually trains better.

Why Random Workouts Can Reinforce the Problem

Random workouts can make you tired. They can make you sweat. They can even make you stronger in some ways.

But random workouts do not always rebuild structure.

If a program never checks your posture, mobility, control, or readiness, it may keep feeding the same patterns you already have.

If your right side always dominates, a random workout may let it keep dominating. If your low back always takes over, a random workout may let it keep taking over. If your shoulders always shrug during upper-body work, a random workout may make that pattern stronger. If your knees cave in during lower-body training, a random workout may load that pattern again and again.

The body gets better at what it repeats.

That is the blessing and the warning.

If you repeat better structure, you can build better strength. If you repeat compensation, you can build stronger compensation.

That is why structure-first training is not about doing more exercises. It is about choosing the right starting point.

The DominionBuilt Sequence

The structure-first path follows a clear order:

Position → Control → Load → Capacity

Position comes first. Can the body find a better starting point?

Control comes second. Can the body own the movement?

Load comes third. Can the body tolerate resistance without losing the pattern?

Capacity comes fourth. Can the body repeat the work, recover from it, and build over time?

Most people want to start at load. They want the workout. They want the program. They want the intensity. They want the result.

But after 40, skipping the earlier steps often costs more than it saves.

Position without control is fragile. Control without load is incomplete. Load without capacity becomes breakdown. Capacity without structure is limited.

Each step matters.

This does not mean you need to spend months doing nothing but corrective drills. It means your training should respect the order.

You can build strength while improving structure. But you cannot ignore structure and expect strength to stay clean forever.

WHAT THIS EXPLAINS

If you have been training consistently but still feel stuck, this may explain why. Your effort may be real. But your structure may not be supporting the work.

If certain exercises always bother the same areas, this may explain why. The exercise may be exposing a position, control, or mobility issue.

If one side always feels stronger, this may explain why. Your body may have built a strategy that favors one side because it feels safer or more familiar.

If you feel tight after every workout, this may explain why. Your body may be protecting itself from positions it does not fully control.

If you can lift more weight but feel worse over time, this may explain why. You may be increasing load faster than your structure can handle.

If you keep starting over, this may explain why. You may not be failing because of motivation. You may be missing the foundation that makes consistency easier to sustain.

The Shift From Effort to Structure

Effort is still necessary. Nothing in this book replaces discipline.

You still have to show up. You still have to move. You still have to practice. You still have to build strength over time.

But effort needs direction.

A body over 40 does not need punishment. It needs a plan. It needs assessment. It needs better positions. It needs usable mobility. It needs stability. It needs strength built in the right order.

This is the shift:

From random effort to structure. From pushing through to paying attention. From chasing workouts to reading patterns. From forcing strength to building capacity.

Your body is not asking you to stop getting stronger. It is asking you to build strength on something it can trust.

That is why structure governs strength.

And now that you understand the principle, we need to look at what happens when structure breaks down across the body.

That is where compensation begins.

CHAPTER 3

The Compensation Chain

The compensation chain is easiest to see in a movement that should be simple. Someone reaches overhead to get something off a high shelf. The arm goes up, the ribcage lifts, the lower back arches, and the neck tightens to make the reach feel complete. From the outside it looks fine. But three structures just did the work of one. The shoulder reached, but the ribs, low back, and neck all helped. That is not a shoulder problem. That is a compensation chain running through four regions because one of them stopped contributing well enough to do the job alone.

The body is connected.

That sounds simple. But most people do not train, stretch, or think that way. They think in parts.

My neck is tight. My shoulder hurts. My back is stiff. My hips are locked. My knees bother me. My feet feel unstable. My core feels weak.

Each area gets treated like a separate problem. So the neck gets stretched. The shoulder gets strengthened. The back gets rested. The hips get opened. The knees get protected. The feet get ignored. The core gets trained harder.

Sometimes that helps. But sometimes the same problems return because the body was never read as a system.

A tight neck may not start in the neck. A sore low back may not start in the low back. A knee problem may not start in the knee. A weak glute may not only be a glute problem.

The area that speaks the loudest is not always the area that started the conversation.

That is why compensation matters.

Compensation is the body's way of getting the job done when one area cannot do its part well. It is not always bad. Sometimes compensation is protective. Sometimes it helps you keep moving. Sometimes it helps you get through a season.

But when compensation becomes your normal pattern, the body starts paying a price.

That price may show up as stiffness, weakness, irritation, uneven strength, poor mobility, low confidence, or the feeling that your body is always working around something.

This is the compensation chain. And once you understand it, your body starts making more sense.

What Compensation Means

Compensation means one area of the body is doing extra work because another area is limited, unstable, weak, restricted, or poorly controlled.

It is the body's workaround system.

If your ankle does not move well, your knee or hip may adjust. If your hips do not extend well, your low back may arch more. If your upper back does not rotate well, your neck or low back may rotate instead. If your core does not stabilize well, your body may create tension in the low back, hip flexors, shoulders, or neck. If your feet do not create a stable base, your knees and hips may shift to help you balance.

The body is smart. It wants to complete the task. If one area cannot contribute well, another area often steps in.

At first, that may feel like success. You still walked. You still lifted. You still climbed the stairs. You still finished the workout.

But over time, the body may become efficient at the wrong strategy. That is where the problem begins.

Because the body gets better at what it repeats. If it repeats better structure, it can build better capacity. If it repeats compensation, it can build stronger compensation.

And strong compensation can feel like strength for a while. Until it starts to feel like breakdown.

The Body Borrows Movement

When one area lacks mobility, the body often borrows movement from somewhere else.

This is one of the most common reasons people feel stiff, tight, or beat up after 40. The body is trying to complete a movement with limited options.

For example, if your upper back is stiff, your shoulder may not move as freely. So when you reach overhead, your neck may tighten, your low back may arch, or your ribs may flare to help you get the arm up.

If your hips are stiff, your low back may help you bend, rotate, or extend. You may think your back is the problem. But the back may be doing extra work because the hips are not giving you enough range.

If your ankles are limited, your squat pattern may change. Your heels may lift. Your knees may shift. Your hips may tuck. Your torso may fold forward.

Borrowed movement is not always painful at first. That is why it can go unnoticed. The body can hide compensation for a long time.

But eventually, the area that keeps lending motion may get tired of paying the bill.

That is when the signal shows up. Tightness. Irritation. Weakness. Guarding. Uneven movement. A pattern that keeps returning.

The question is not only: Where do I feel it?

The better question is: What is my body borrowing to make this movement happen?

The Body Borrows Stability

The body does not only borrow movement. It also borrows stability.

When one area does not feel supported, another area may tighten to create a sense of control.

This is why some people feel tight all the time even though they stretch. The tightness may not be a flexibility issue. It may be a stability strategy.

If your core does not organize well, your low back may tighten to create support. If your shoulder blade does not control well, your neck and traps may grip during upper-body movement. If your hip lacks stability, your knee may feel less secure. If your foot does not create stable contact with the floor, your whole lower body may feel uncertain.

The body likes safety. If it does not feel safe through control, it may create safety through tension.

That tension can feel like tightness. But if you only stretch the tight area, the body may tighten again because the stability problem was never addressed.

This is why a structure-first approach does not chase every tight muscle. It asks why the tightness keeps coming back.

Is the area short? Or is it guarding? Is it restricted? Or is it protecting? Is it weak? Or is it overworked?

Those questions matter. Because the answer changes the solution.

The Body Borrows Strength

Sometimes the body borrows strength from the wrong areas.

This is why certain exercises do not feel the way they are supposed to feel.

A glute exercise goes to the hamstrings. A core exercise goes to the low back. A shoulder exercise goes to the neck. A leg exercise goes to the knees. A back exercise goes to the biceps or traps.

The body completes the movement, but the wrong area carries the load.

Again, this does not mean the exercise is bad. It may mean your body does not yet have the position, control, or connection needed to access the intended muscle well.

For example, if your pelvis is not organized well, your glutes may not contribute the way you expect. If your ribs flare and your low back arches during core work, your trunk may not stabilize the way you need. If your shoulders sit forward and your upper back is stiff, your neck may become too involved during pressing, pulling, or reaching.

This is why better structure often improves muscle connection. The muscle did not suddenly appear. The body simply found a better pathway to use it.

That is the goal. Not to force every muscle. Not to chase soreness. But to improve the structure so strength can show up where it belongs.

The Three Regions DominionBuilt Reads

To keep this simple, DominionBuilt looks at the body through three major regions:

Upper Chain. Core Stack. Base.

These are not separate systems. They are connected layers. But separating them helps you see the chain more clearly.

The upper chain includes the head, neck, shoulders, and upper back.

The core stack includes the ribcage, pelvis, spine, breathing, and trunk control.

The base includes the hips, knees, feet, stance, balance, and gait.

Each region can affect the others. A forward head and rounded shoulders can change how the ribcage sits. A poor ribcage and pelvis relationship can change how the hips and core work. Weak foot pressure or poor hip control can change how the knees, pelvis, and low back respond.

This is why the body has to be read in layers. Not because every problem is complicated. But because the body is connected.

The goal is not to create fear or overanalysis. The goal is to stop treating every symptom like an isolated event.

Why the Painful Area Is Not Always the Source

This is one of the most important ideas in the book:

The painful area is not always the source.

Sometimes it is. If you have a specific injury, trauma, swelling, sharp pain, numbness, tingling, or symptoms that concern you, you should seek qualified care.

But in many movement patterns, the area that complains may be the area that is overworked, not the area that started the problem.

The low back may complain because the hips are not moving well. The neck may complain because the upper back is stiff and the shoulders are poorly positioned. The knees may complain because the hips and feet are not controlling force. The shoulders may complain because the ribcage and upper back are not giving them a good platform.

This is why chasing pain can become frustrating. You stretch the back, but the hips are still locked. You massage the neck, but the upper back still does not move. You protect the knee, but the foot and hip pattern never changes. You rest the shoulder, but the ribcage and shoulder blade mechanics stay the same.

A structure-first approach asks: What is this area doing? What is it compensating for? What is above it? What is below it? What is the pattern?

That is how you begin to read the chain.

How Compensation Travels

Compensation can travel up or down the body.

A foot problem can affect the knee. A knee strategy can affect the hip. A hip limitation can affect the low back. A ribcage position can affect the shoulder. A stiff upper back can affect the neck. A weak trunk can affect almost everything.

This does not mean every issue causes every other issue. The body is not that simple. But it does mean movement is connected.

The chain is not always dramatic. Sometimes it is subtle. But subtle patterns repeated for years can become loud later.

That is why compensation has to be respected.

The Goal Is Not Perfection

Reading the compensation chain does not mean you need perfect posture. It does not mean every movement has to look textbook. It does not mean you should become afraid of every small asymmetry.

No human body is perfectly symmetrical. No movement is perfectly clean all the time. No structure is flawless.

The goal is not perfection. The goal is awareness.

Can you see the pattern? Can you identify where the body is borrowing too much? Can you tell when the same area keeps taking over? Can you notice when tightness keeps returning? Can you tell when load is being added to poor control? Can you begin choosing better starting points?

That is the work. Not obsessing. Not diagnosing yourself. Not becoming afraid of movement. Just learning how to listen with more structure.

The First Layer of the Map

Now you have the first layer of the map.

Your body is connected. Your symptoms may be connected. Your strength is connected to structure. Your structure is affected by the upper chain, the core stack, and the base.

When one area loses position, mobility, or control, another area may compensate. That compensation may help for a while. But if it becomes your normal pattern, it can eventually create restriction, irritation, weakness, or loss of confidence.

This is not a reason to panic. It is a reason to pay attention.

Because once you can see the chain, you can begin to reset it.

The next step is to look more closely at the first major region:

The Upper Chain.

Your head, neck, shoulders, and upper back carry more of your movement story than you may realize.

Part Two

Reading the Body

CHAPTER 4

The Upper Chain: Why Your Neck, Shoulders, and Upper Back Feel Tight

A person in their late 40s has been training for years. Not sedentary — genuinely committed. But their overhead press has become restricted and their lower back takes over on rows. Their neck tightens on carries. Their shoulders shrug on pulls instead of pulling from the back. Three different movements, three different compensation patterns, all running through the same chain. The upper back stopped extending and rotating well, so the neck and traps took over. Nothing is torn. The chain reorganized around a stiffness it learned to work around rather than through.

This chapter explains how that chain is organized, why each area affects the others, and where the reset work needs to begin.

Modern life pulls the upper body forward.

Not all at once. Slowly. Hour by hour. Day by day. Year by year.

You sit at a desk. You drive. You look down at your phone. You carry stress in your shoulders. You reach forward more than you reach overhead. You breathe shallow. You train around stiffness instead of addressing it.

Then one day your upper body starts to feel different. Your neck feels tight. Your shoulders sit forward. Your upper back feels locked. Your traps always seem tense. Reaching overhead feels harder than it should. Pressing feels awkward. Pulling does not feel clean.

You stretch your neck, roll your shoulders, massage your traps, and maybe it helps for a little while. But the tightness comes back.

That is when you need to look deeper. Because the issue may not be one tight muscle. It may be the upper chain.

At DominionBuilt, the upper chain includes:

head

neck

shoulders

shoulder blades

upper back

chest position

ribcage relationship

These areas work together. When one part of the upper chain loses position, mobility, or control, another part often compensates.

The body is connected. And the upper chain is one of the clearest places to see that connection.

What Happens When the Upper Body Drifts Forward

The body is designed to adapt. If you spend enough time in a position, your body starts treating that position as normal. That is useful when the position supports you. It becomes a problem when the position limits you.

Many adults over 40 spend years in a forward-dominant posture. The head drifts forward. The shoulders round. The upper back stiffens. The chest tightens. The shoulder blades lose clean movement. The ribs may stay lifted. The neck and traps start doing work they were never meant to carry all day.

This does not mean your posture has to be perfect. It does not mean you need to walk around stiff and upright all day.

The issue is not one posture. The issue is losing options.

You should be able to round. You should be able to extend. You should be able to rotate. You should be able to reach. You should be able to breathe. You should be able to move the shoulders without the neck taking over.

When the upper body gets stuck in one dominant position, movement becomes more expensive. The body can still perform. But it has fewer options. And fewer options usually means more compensation.

Forward Head Position

Forward head position is one of the most common upper-chain patterns. The head drifts in front of the body instead of resting more directly over the ribcage.

When this happens, the neck has to work harder. Your head is not light. When it moves forward, the muscles around the neck and upper back often create more tension to hold it there.

Over time, this can contribute to tightness, fatigue, headaches, trap tension, or that constant feeling that your neck needs to be stretched.

The mistake is trying to fix this by only stretching the neck. Stretching may feel good. But if the head keeps returning to the same forward position, the body will keep asking the neck to carry the same load.

The better question is: Why does my head keep living there?

It may connect to your upper back. It may connect to your ribcage. It may connect to breathing. It may connect to shoulder position. It may connect to your daily habits.

The neck is often the messenger. Not always the root.

Rounded Shoulders

Rounded shoulders are another common upper-chain pattern. This is when the shoulders sit forward and the chest appears collapsed or shortened.

This is not about shaming posture. It is about function.

If the shoulders live forward for long enough, the body may lose strength and control in the muscles that help position the shoulder blades. Pressing, pulling, reaching, and carrying can all feel different.

This matters because the shoulder is not just the shoulder joint. The shoulder depends on the shoulder blade. The shoulder blade depends on the ribcage. The ribcage depends on trunk position and breathing.

This is why simply pulling your shoulders back is not a real solution. That usually creates tension. It does not create better control.

A better goal is to restore the shoulder's ability to move, sit, and stabilize with less compensation. You do not need forced posture. You need usable position.

Upper-Back Stiffness

The upper back, also called the thoracic spine, plays a major role in how the upper body moves. It helps you extend, rotate, reach, breathe, position the shoulders, and transfer force through the trunk.

When the upper back gets stiff, other areas often compensate. The neck may move more. The low back may arch more. The shoulders may lose clean motion. The ribs may flare. Breathing may become shallow.

A stiff upper back can make the whole upper chain feel older than it should. And after years of sitting, driving, screen time, stress, and limited rotation, this pattern is common.

The answer is not aggressive forcing. The answer is restoring movement gradually. The upper back needs to learn how to move again without the neck or low back doing all the work.

Tight Traps and Neck Tension

Many people over 40 feel like their traps are always tight. They stretch them. Massage them. Roll them. Dig into them. And still, the tension returns.

That is because traps often tighten for a reason. Sometimes they are overworked because the shoulders are poorly positioned. Sometimes they are helping the neck hold a forward head posture. Sometimes they are compensating for weak or poorly controlled shoulder blades. Sometimes shallow breathing keeps the upper chest and neck more active than they need to be. Sometimes stress lives there.

The body does not separate emotional tension and physical tension as neatly as people think.

If the traps are always tight, do not only ask: How do I stretch them? Ask: Why are they always being asked to work?

That question changes the direction. The tight area is speaking. But you still have to understand the message.

Why Desk Life Affects Training

A lot of people separate their workouts from the rest of their day. They think: I train for one hour. That should fix it.

But your body does not only adapt to the workout. It adapts to the other twenty-three hours too.

If you sit for long periods with your head forward, shoulders rounded, ribs compressed, and hips tucked or locked, then walk into the gym and ask your body to press, pull, hinge, squat, run, or rotate, your body brings that posture history with it.

The workout does not erase the day. Sometimes it exposes the day.

If your upper back has been rounded all day, overhead movement may feel restricted. If your neck has been working all day, shoulder training may create more tension. If your ribcage has been compressed, breathing and bracing may feel harder. If your shoulders have been forward all day, pressing may feel awkward.

Training does not happen in a vacuum. Your structure comes with you.

When the Shoulder Takes the Blame

The shoulder often gets blamed for upper-chain problems. Shoulder discomfort is common, shoulder movement is complex, and when it does not feel right, it can affect almost every upper-body exercise.

But the shoulder is often downstream from other patterns.

The shoulder joint depends on the shoulder blade. The shoulder blade sits on the ribcage. The ribcage is influenced by breathing, trunk position, and upper-back mobility. If those pieces are not working well, the shoulder may not have the platform it needs.

A shoulder that feels weak or irritated may need shoulder work. But it may also need better upper-back movement, ribcage control, breathing, and shoulder blade mechanics.

This is why structure-first training does not rush to isolate one area too quickly. It asks: What does the shoulder need from the rest of the chain?

The Upper Chain and Breathing

Many people do not connect breathing with the upper body. But the connection is real.

When breathing is shallow, the neck and upper chest often help lift the ribcage. Over time, the muscles around the neck, shoulders, and upper ribs may stay more active than they need to be. This can feed tension.

When the ribs stay flared or lifted, the shoulder blades may not sit as well on the ribcage. When the ribcage does not move well, the upper back and shoulders may lose options.

This is why breathing is not just relaxation. It is structure. Breathing does not fix everything. But it is one piece of the upper-chain map. And it is often overlooked.

Self-Check 1: Wall Posture Check

This is not a diagnosis. It is awareness.

Stand with your back near a wall. Place your heels a few inches away from the wall. Let your hips, upper back, and head move toward the wall naturally. Do not force anything. Do not jam your head back. Do not overarch your low back. Just notice.

Can the back of your head reach the wall without strain? Do your ribs flare up to make it happen? Do you feel your low back arch hard? Do your shoulders feel like they are pulled forward? Do you feel tension in your neck?

This check gives you information about your resting posture. If your head cannot reach the wall comfortably, that may suggest forward head position or upper-back stiffness. If your ribs flare or low back arches, your body may be borrowing from the lower back to create the position.

Do not judge it. Just notice it. The goal is not to pass the check. The goal is to learn what your body is showing you.

Takeaway: If this feels restricted or strained, your upper chain may need better position, mobility, or control before heavier pressing or overhead work.

Self-Check 2: Shoulder Reach Check

Stand tall or sit upright. Reach both arms overhead slowly. Do not force the movement. Notice what happens.

Can your arms reach overhead without your low back arching? Do your ribs flare? Do your shoulders shrug toward your ears? Do you feel pinching, restriction, or tension? Does one side move easier than the other? Can you breathe while holding the position?

This check helps you see how your shoulders, upper back, ribcage, and trunk work together. If your shoulders cannot reach overhead without compensation, the issue may not only be shoulder flexibility. It may involve upper-back mobility, rib position, breathing, shoulder blade control, or trunk stability.

This is not a diagnosis. It is direction.

Takeaway: If reaching overhead makes your ribs flare, neck tighten, or low back arch, your body may be borrowing motion instead of owning the position.

Self-Check 3: Upper-Back Rotation Check

Sit tall in a chair. Cross your arms gently over your chest. Keep your hips facing forward. Slowly rotate your upper body to one side. Then rotate to the other side. Do not force. Do not twist aggressively. Notice the difference.

Does one side feel more restricted? Do your shoulders move with you? Do you feel the rotation in your upper back, or do you feel it mostly in your low back? Can you breathe while rotating?

Upper-back rotation matters for reaching, walking, turning, pressing, pulling, and many daily movements. If the upper back does not rotate well, the neck, shoulders, or low back may borrow movement.

The goal is not extreme range. The goal is controlled movement without strain.

Takeaway: If rotation feels limited or uneven, your upper back may need more usable movement before your shoulders and neck can fully relax.

Self-Check 4: Neck Position Awareness

Sit or stand normally. Do not correct anything yet. Notice where your head naturally rests. Is your chin lifted? Is your chin tucked down? Is your head drifting forward? Do you feel tension at the base of your skull? Are your shoulders relaxed, or are they slightly elevated?

Now gently imagine your head floating upward from the crown. Let the back of your neck lengthen slightly. Do not force a hard chin tuck. Do not stiffen. Just create a little more space.

Can you breathe there? Does it feel natural or strange?

A better neck position should feel supported, not forced.

Takeaway: If a gentle position change feels difficult to maintain, your neck may be compensating for upper-chain position, breathing, or shoulder tension.

First Steps to Reset the Upper Chain

The goal is not to fix everything in one day. The goal is to begin giving your body better signals.

These are not full programs yet. They are reset categories.

A true upper-chain reset may include:

breathing with rib awareness

gentle upper-back movement

shoulder blade control

wall posture awareness

controlled overhead reach

light pulling patterns with good position

None of this has to be extreme. In fact, it should not be.

The upper chain often responds well to consistency, not force. You are teaching the body that it has options again. That it does not have to live forward all day. That the neck does not have to do everything. That the shoulders can move from a better platform. That the upper back can contribute again.

That is the reset.

The Upper Chain Is the First Window

The upper chain is often the first place people notice their body changing after 40. The neck gets tight. The shoulders round. The upper back stiffens. Training starts feeling different. Posture changes slowly.

But once you understand the upper chain, you can stop treating every tight muscle like a separate problem. You can start reading the structure.

Head position. Shoulder position. Upper-back mobility. Ribcage relationship. Breathing. Control. These are all part of the same conversation.

The next layer is even deeper. Because beneath the upper chain is the center that connects everything above and below.

That is where we go next:

The Core Stack.

CHAPTER 5

The Core Stack: Why Your Back Takes Over

Someone in their mid-40s has persistent low-back tension. They have strengthened the core, stretched the hip flexors, and tried every back exercise their program includes. The tension keeps returning within hours of training. What the assessment reveals is that the ribcage has been sitting in a lifted position for so long that the lumbar spine is doing stability work that belongs to the trunk. The pelvis cannot find neutral because the ribs will not come down. The low-back tension is the result, not the problem.

Addressing the ribcage and pelvis position first — before loading anything else — is often the difference between training that builds and training that keeps producing the same complaint.

Most people think the core means abs.

They think of crunches, planks, sit-ups, twists, and the visible muscles around the waist. That is part of the picture. But it is not the whole picture.

Your core is not just a muscle group. It is the center of your structure. It is where your ribcage, pelvis, spine, breathing, and trunk control all meet.

When that center is organized well, your body has a better platform for movement. Your shoulders can move from a more stable base. Your hips can produce force with better control. Your low back does not have to do every job. Your breathing can support movement instead of fighting against it.

But when the core stack is poorly organized, the body often finds another way. That "other way" is usually tension. The low back tightens. The hip flexors grip. The ribs flare. The pelvis tips. The breath gets shallow. The body feels braced even when you are not training.

And eventually, you may start saying things like: "My back always takes over." "My core feels weak no matter what I do." "I feel tight through my hips and low back." "I do core exercises, but I never really feel my core." "I can lift, but I do not feel stable."

That is when you need to look at the core stack. Not just the abs. The whole center.

At DominionBuilt, the core stack includes:

ribcage

pelvis

spine

breathing

trunk control

bracing

how the upper body and lower body connect

The core stack is the bridge. It connects the upper chain to the base.

If the bridge is unstable, stiff, collapsed, overarched, or poorly controlled, everything above and below it has to adjust. That is why the low back often takes over.

Your Core Is More Than Abs

A strong-looking midsection does not always mean a well-functioning core.

Someone can have visible abs and still struggle to brace well. Someone can hold a plank and still overuse their low back. Someone can do hundreds of crunches and still feel unstable during squats, hinges, lunges, presses, or daily movement.

That is because the core is not only about contraction. It is about organization.

Can your ribcage and pelvis relate well? Can your spine maintain position under effort? Can you breathe without losing control? Can you create tension when needed and release tension when it is no longer needed? Can your trunk transfer force between your upper body and lower body? Can you move your arms and legs without your low back becoming the main stabilizer?

That is core function. The goal is not to squeeze your abs all day. The goal is to create a body that can stabilize, breathe, rotate, resist motion, transfer force, and move with control.

That is why random core exercises often fail. They train effort. But they do not always train organization.

The Ribcage and Pelvis Relationship

The ribcage and pelvis are two major anchors of your structure. When they work together, the trunk has a clearer center. When they are disconnected, the body often compensates.

One common pattern is the ribs flaring upward while the pelvis tips forward. This can make the low back arch more than it should.

Another pattern is the pelvis tucking under too much. This can flatten the low back, reduce hip access, and make movement feel restricted or guarded.

Neither position is automatically "bad" in every moment. The body should be able to move through different positions. The problem is when one position becomes the default and the body loses options.

If the ribs and pelvis do not stack well, the trunk may struggle to stabilize. When the trunk struggles to stabilize, the low back may work overtime. That is why the low back often becomes the place people feel everything.

Rib Flare

Rib flare happens when the lower ribs lift or widen forward instead of staying more connected to the rest of the trunk.

It can affect how the body stabilizes. When the ribs stay lifted, the abs may not connect as well. The diaphragm and deep trunk muscles may not coordinate as cleanly. The low back may become the place that creates the missing support.

The goal is not to clamp the ribs. The goal is awareness and control. Can you bring the ribs into a better relationship with the pelvis? Can you breathe there? Can you move there? Can you create effort there without the low back taking over?

Pelvic Position

The pelvis is another major part of the core stack. If it tips forward too much, the low back may arch, the hip flexors may feel tight, and the glutes may be harder to access. If it tucks under too much, the hips may feel restricted and movement may lose power.

Many adults over 40 lose awareness of pelvic position. They do not know when they are overarched. They do not know when they are tucked. They do not know why their low back tightens during exercises that are supposed to train the legs, glutes, or core.

If you cannot feel where your pelvis is, it is harder to control what your trunk and hips are doing. And if the pelvis is poorly controlled, the low back often becomes the backup plan.

Why Breathing Matters

Breathing is one of the most overlooked parts of structure. You breathe all day. But not all breathing supports movement well.

Shallow breathing often keeps the upper chest, neck, and shoulders more active. Poor exhaling can leave the ribs lifted and the trunk poorly organized. Holding your breath too much can create tension without control. Breathing poorly under effort can make exercise feel harder than it needs to be.

A good exhale can help bring the ribs and pelvis into a better relationship. A better inhale can help the ribcage expand instead of staying locked. Better breathing can reduce unnecessary tension and improve awareness of the trunk.

If you cannot breathe in a position, your body may not trust that position. If you lose your breath every time a movement gets hard, your structure may not be organized enough to support the effort.

The core stack is not separate from breathing. Breathing is part of how the stack works.

Why the Low Back Takes Over

The low back often takes over when the rest of the core stack is not doing its job well enough.

It may happen because the ribs are flared. It may happen because the pelvis is tipped forward. It may happen because the hips are restricted. It may happen because the trunk does not brace well. It may happen because the glutes are not contributing. It may happen because the person is using load before control.

The low back is not the villain. It is often the helper that got overused. It steps in when the body needs stability, helps when the hips do not move well, supports when the core does not organize well, and tightens when the body feels unsafe.

The problem is that the low back was not designed to carry every job. If it keeps taking over, the body may start to feel guarded, stiff, irritated, or unreliable.

Why Core Training Often Misses the Point

Many people respond to low-back tightness or weak-core feelings by doing more core exercises. More planks. More crunches. More sit-ups. More leg raises. More twists.

Some of those exercises may have value. But they do not automatically fix the core stack.

A plank can still be done with rib flare. A sit-up can still reinforce hip flexor dominance. A leg raise can still pull the low back into extension. A crunch can still train effort without teaching control.

A structure-first approach does not ask: "How many core exercises can I do?" It asks: "Can my body organize the center well enough to support movement?"

That question changes everything.

The Core Stack and the Hips

The core stack affects the hips more than many people realize. If the pelvis is poorly positioned or poorly controlled, the hips may not move well. If the ribs and pelvis are disconnected, the glutes may not contribute cleanly.

This is why hip tightness often connects to the core stack. A person may stretch the hip flexors repeatedly and feel relief for a few minutes. Then the tightness comes back.

That does not always mean the stretch was wrong. It may mean the body still lacks the trunk and pelvic control needed to keep the hip from guarding again.

When the center improves, hip movement often has a better chance to improve too.

The Core Stack and the Shoulders

The core stack also affects the shoulders. The shoulder blade sits on the ribcage. If the ribcage is poorly positioned, the shoulder blade may not move or stabilize as well. If the trunk cannot stabilize during pressing or pulling, the shoulders may feel less supported.

When the core stack is better organized, the shoulders often have a better platform. That gives the upper chain a stronger foundation.

Self-Check 1: Rib-Pelvis Stack Check

This is not a diagnosis. It is awareness.

Stand sideways in front of a mirror if possible. Place one hand lightly on your lower ribs. Place the other hand on the front of your pelvis. Notice the relationship.

Are your ribs lifted high? Does your low back feel arched? Does your pelvis feel tipped forward?

Now gently exhale. Let the ribs soften down slightly without collapsing. Imagine the ribcage and pelvis facing each other more directly. Do not squeeze hard. Do not force. Just notice whether you can find a more stacked position.

Can you breathe there? Can you stand there without tension?

Takeaway: If stacking your ribs and pelvis feels difficult, your low back may be helping create posture instead of your trunk organizing the position.

Self-Check 2: Breathing Check

Lie on your back with your knees bent, or sit tall in a chair. Place one hand on your upper chest. Place one hand around the lower ribs or belly. Take a slow breath in.

Does your chest rise first? Do your shoulders lift? Do your neck muscles tighten? Do your lower ribs move at all?

Now exhale slowly. Can you feel your ribs come down slightly? Can you exhale without clenching? Can you breathe without your shoulders doing most of the work?

Takeaway: If every breath lifts your chest, neck, or shoulders, your breathing may be feeding tension instead of helping organize the core stack.

Self-Check 3: Brace Awareness Drill

Stand tall or sit upright. Place your hands around your waist. Take a calm breath in. Exhale slightly. Now imagine preparing your trunk as if someone were about to gently push your side.

Do not suck in. Do not bear down aggressively. Do not hold your breath. Create firm, even tension around the trunk.

Can you breathe while maintaining that tension? Can you keep your ribs from flaring? Can you avoid gripping your low back? Can you keep your shoulders relaxed?

Takeaway: If bracing makes you hold your breath, arch your back, or tighten your neck, your body may need better trunk control before heavier loading.

Self-Check 4: Standing Low-Back Awareness

Stand normally. Do not correct anything yet. Notice your low back. Does it feel relaxed? Does it feel arched? Does it feel clenched? Do your ribs feel lifted? Do your hip flexors feel tight?

Now gently shift your pelvis forward and backward. Find the extremes. Then settle near the middle. Let your ribs soften slightly. Take a slow breath.

Can your low back relax a little without you collapsing? Can you stand with less tension?

Takeaway: If your low back feels constantly active even while standing still, it may be compensating for poor rib-pelvis organization, hip position, or trunk control.

First Steps to Reset the Core Stack

The goal is not to brace harder all day. The goal is to create better awareness, better breathing, and better control.

Start simple. Learn where your ribs are. Learn where your pelvis is. Learn how you breathe. Learn how to create tension without gripping. Learn how to move your arms and legs while the center stays organized.

These are reset categories, not a full program yet. A true core-stack reset may include:

breathing with rib awareness

gentle exhale practice

rib-pelvis stacking

low-back tension awareness

beginner core stability

controlled arm and leg movement

glute activation with trunk control

You are not trying to crush your core. You are teaching your body how to organize the middle again.

The Core Stack Is the Bridge

The upper chain gave you the first window. Now the core stack gives you the bridge.

It connects what happens above with what happens below. The center affects both ends. That is why your low back may take over. That is why your hips may feel tight. That is why your shoulders may feel unsupported. That is why strength may feel unstable.

The core stack is not about chasing abs. It is about building a center your body can trust.

And once you understand the center, the next step is to look at the foundation beneath it.

That is where we go next:

The Base.

CHAPTER 6

The Base: Why Your Hips, Knees, and Feet Control More Than You Think

---

Three different people, same pattern: the lower body limiting the upper body. A runner whose knee loads more than it should on longer efforts, despite consistent hip flexor and IT band work. A parent who gets off the floor awkwardly now and has to think about it. A lifter whose squat depth has quietly disappeared without any injury explaining it. In all three cases, the base stopped contributing and the chain above reorganized around that loss. Starting at the foundation changed what the rest of the chain could do.

The body is built from the ground up.

That does not mean every problem starts in the feet. It means your base matters.

Your hips, knees, ankles, feet, stance, balance, and walking pattern all affect how the rest of your body moves. If your base is strong, stable, mobile, and well controlled, your body has something to build from. If your base is restricted, unstable, uneven, or poorly controlled, the body starts making adjustments.

The knees may take more stress. The hips may tighten. The low back may work harder. Balance may feel less reliable. Lower-body exercises may feel awkward.

And after 40, many people begin noticing this first in daily life. Getting up from a chair feels harder. Going downstairs feels less confident. One hip feels tighter than the other. One knee complains more than the other. Your feet feel less stable. Your balance feels less automatic. Your stride feels shorter. You avoid positions you used to move through without thinking.

That is not always because your body is broken. It may be because your base has lost some of the mobility, control, strength, and confidence it used to have.

At DominionBuilt, the base includes:

hips

knees

ankles

feet

stance

balance

gait

lower-body control

The base is your contact point with the ground. It is how force enters the body. It is how strength moves through the body. It is how your body supports posture, motion, and training. If the base is not working well, the rest of the structure has to compensate.

The Hips Drive Movement

The hips are one of the most important areas in the body. They affect walking, standing, squatting, hinging, climbing stairs, getting up from the floor, rotating, balancing, carrying, and training.

When the hips move well, the body usually has more options. When the hips are restricted, the body often borrows from somewhere else. The low back may move more. The knees may take more stress. The feet may shift. The pelvis may tilt or rotate. The trunk may lean.

The hips are not just a lower-body issue. They are part of the whole structure. When the hips do not contribute well, other areas often pay.

Hip Mobility and Hip Control

Hip mobility matters. But mobility alone is not enough. You also need control.

If the hip can move into a range but cannot control that range, the body may still guard. If the hip cannot move into a range at all, the body may borrow from the low back, knees, or feet.

The hip needs usable mobility. That means the joint can access range, control the range, and use the range during real movement.

The goal is not endless stretching. The goal is controlled movement. The hip must learn to open, rotate, stabilize, and produce force without forcing another area to take over.

Glute Control and the Base

The glutes help extend the hip, stabilize the pelvis, control the femur, and support walking, climbing, lifting, squatting, hinging, and standing.

When the glutes do not contribute well, the body may find other ways to complete the task. The hamstrings may overwork. The low back may tighten. The hip flexors may grip. The knees may feel more stress.

You cannot force a muscle to do its job well if the structure keeps giving the job to another area. The goal is not just glute activation. The goal is better lower-body organization.

The Knees Reveal the Chain

The knee sits between the hip and the foot. That means it is influenced from above and below.

If the hip cannot control rotation well, the knee may drift. If the foot collapses or loses pressure, the knee may shift. If the ankle lacks mobility, the knee may compensate. If the glute is not helping, the knee may take more load.

Structure-first thinking asks: What is the knee responding to?

The knee reveals the chain. It often tells you whether the hip, foot, ankle, and trunk are coordinating well enough.

Foot Pressure Matters

Your feet are your first connection to the ground. Every step, squat, lunge, hinge, and carry begins with ground contact. If the feet are not creating stable pressure, the rest of the body has to adjust.

A useful concept is the foot tripod. That means feeling pressure through three points:

base of the big toe

base of the little toe

heel

When those three points connect to the ground, the foot often creates a more stable platform. That platform can help the knee track better, the hip respond better, balance improve, and strength feel more grounded.

Balance Is a Strength Skill

Balance is a strength skill. It is a nervous system skill. It is a control skill. It is a confidence skill.

After 40, balance can quietly decline if it is not trained or challenged. You may notice it when standing on one leg, stepping off a curb, walking on uneven ground, or going downstairs.

Loss of balance can make people move smaller. They stop using certain ranges. They avoid certain exercises. They become less confident. Then the base loses even more capacity.

A stronger base is not only about lifting more weight. It is about being able to control your body when life asks for it.

Gait: The Pattern You Repeat Most

Walking is one of the most repeated movements in your life. Gait is just the pattern of how you walk. It includes your feet, ankles, knees, hips, pelvis, trunk, arms, and rhythm.

Walking can reveal a lot. Do you shift more to one side? Does one foot turn out? Do your arms swing evenly? Do your hips rotate? Do you feel one side working harder?

Walking is not just cardio. It is a structure pattern repeated thousands of times. If the pattern is efficient, walking can support your body. If the pattern is uneven or compensatory, walking may reinforce the same issues every day.

Self-Check 1: Stance Check

Stand naturally. Do not correct anything yet. Look down at your feet. Are they pointed straight ahead, turned out, or turned in? Is one foot different from the other? Do you feel more weight on one side?

Now gently find your foot tripod. Feel the base of the big toe, the base of the little toe, and the heel. Try to create steady pressure through all three points. Do not force your arches. Do not claw the floor.

Takeaway: If your stance feels uneven or hard to control, your base may need better foot awareness before harder lower-body training.

Self-Check 2: Single-Leg Balance Check

Stand near a wall or stable surface. Shift weight onto one foot. Slowly lift the other foot slightly off the ground. Do not hold your breath. Do not grip your toes. Notice what happens.

Can you balance for ten to twenty seconds? Does one side feel harder? Does your foot collapse or grip? Does your hip shift out to the side? Does your knee wobble? Can you breathe?

Takeaway: If one side feels much less stable, your body may be showing a control difference that strength training should respect.

Self-Check 3: Hip Hinge Check

Stand tall with your feet about hip-width apart. Place your hands on your hips. Keep your spine long. Push your hips back as if closing a car door with your hips. Let your knees bend slightly. Do not squat down. Hinge back. Then return to standing.

Do you feel your hips move back? Do you feel your hamstrings load? Does your low back tighten? Do your knees move forward first?

Takeaway: If your low back takes over during a hinge, your hips, core stack, or foot pressure may need attention before heavier deadlifts or loaded hinging.

Self-Check 4: Squat-to-Chair Check

Stand in front of a chair. Slowly sit back toward the chair. Lightly touch the chair. Then stand back up with control. Do not drop quickly. Do not use momentum.

Do your knees cave inward? Do your heels lift? Does your weight shift to one side? Does your low back round or arch excessively? Do you feel your hips working?

Takeaway: If sitting and standing feels uneven, rushed, or unstable, your base may need more control before higher-intensity lower-body work.

Self-Check 5: Step-Down Awareness Check

Stand on a low step if available. Hold a railing or stable surface. Slowly lower one foot toward the floor. Do not drop. Do not rush. Notice the standing leg.

Does the knee cave inward? Does the foot collapse? Does the hip shift? Does the pelvis drop? Does one side feel different?

Takeaway: If stepping down feels unstable or knee-dominant, your hip, foot, ankle, and quad control may need attention.

First Steps to Reset the Base

The goal is not to force perfect movement. The goal is to restore awareness, stability, and control from the ground up.

These are reset categories, not a full program yet. A true base reset may include:

foot tripod awareness

balance practice

hip mobility

glute control

squat-to-chair practice

hinge patterning

step-down control

walking awareness

You are teaching your body that the ground is safe again. That the hips can move. That the knees can track. That the feet can support. That balance can return. That strength has a foundation.

The Base Gives the Body Confidence

When your feet feel grounded, your body feels more secure. When your hips move better, your low back often has less to borrow. When your knees track better, stairs and lower-body exercises can feel less threatening. When your balance improves, movement feels less risky.

The upper chain gave you the first window. The core stack showed you the bridge. The base shows you the foundation.

Now that you have seen the three major regions, the next step is learning how to stop guessing. Before you push harder, you need to assess what your body is showing you.

That is where we go next:

Assess Before You Push.

CHAPTER 7

Assess Before You Push

Most people start with the workout. They ask: What program should I follow? What exercises should I do? How many days should I train? How much weight should I lift? How hard should I push?

Those questions matter. But they are not the first questions. Not after 40. Not when your body feels stiff, uneven, guarded, weak, or unreliable.

The better first question is:

What is my body showing me?

Because if you do not know what your body is showing you, the workout becomes a guess. You may choose exercises that look right but do not fit your structure. You may stretch areas that are not the real limitation. You may strengthen patterns that are already compensating. You may add load to positions your body does not control. You may push harder when your body actually needs a reset.

This is why assessment matters. Not medical diagnosis. Not fear. Not overanalysis. Assessment.

A structure-first assessment helps you look at your body before you ask more from it. It gives you a starting point, helps you see what needs attention, and helps you stop treating every workout like a random experiment.

At DominionBuilt, the rule is simple:

Assess before you push.

Because the body usually gives signs before it gives bigger warnings. The question is whether you know how to read them.

Why Guessing Creates Frustration

Guessing can feel productive at first. You find a workout online. You try a new routine. You copy exercises that worked for someone else. You add stretching because you feel tight. You add strength because you feel weak. You add intensity because you want results.

Sometimes it helps. But if the workout does not match what your body needs, frustration builds.

You stretch your hips, but they tighten again. You train your core, but your low back still takes over. You work your shoulders, but your neck keeps gripping. You train legs, but your knees feel more involved than your hips. You rest, but nothing really changes. You push, but the body pushes back.

That is the cost of guessing. Not because you lack discipline.

Discipline aimed at the wrong target can still miss.

A structure-first approach does not begin by assuming the problem. It begins by observing the pattern. Where do you lose position? Where do you feel restricted? Where do you feel unstable? Where does one side move differently? Where does tension keep returning? Where does your body borrow from the wrong place?

Those answers help determine the next step. Without them, you may keep working harder without getting clearer.

Assessment Is Not Diagnosis

Assessment is not diagnosis.

A book cannot diagnose your body. A self-check cannot replace a medical evaluation. A posture check cannot tell the whole story.

If you have sharp pain, numbness, tingling, swelling, sudden weakness, unexplained symptoms, trauma, or pain that does not settle, seek qualified care. That is wisdom.

But not every observation is a diagnosis.

There is a difference between saying: "This movement may suggest poor hip control" and saying: "You have a medical condition."

This book is not trying to turn you into your own doctor. It is teaching you to notice patterns. That matters because many people over 40 ignore their body until the signal becomes too loud. Assessment helps you listen earlier. It helps you choose better.

What You Are Looking For

When you assess your body, you are not looking for perfection. You are looking for patterns.

No one moves perfectly. No one is completely symmetrical. No one has flawless posture all day.

Look for five things:

1. Position

2. Mobility

3. Stability

4. Strength pattern

5. Readiness

These five areas give you a simple way to read your body without getting lost. They do not tell you everything. But they give you a starting point. And a better starting point changes everything.

1. Position: Where Does Your Body Start?

Position is your starting point. How do you stand? How do your shoulders sit? Where does your head rest? What does your ribcage do? What does your pelvis do? How do your feet meet the ground?

Position affects the way your body moves before the movement even begins. If your head is forward, your neck may work harder. If your shoulders sit forward, your upper back and shoulder blades may need attention. If your ribs flare, your low back may become more involved. If your pelvis tips forward, your hips and glutes may not contribute cleanly. If your feet collapse or shift, the knees and hips may compensate.

Position does not need to be perfect. But it needs to be understood. A better position gives the body a better chance to produce clean movement. The goal is not forced posture. The goal is usable position.

2. Mobility: What Range Can You Access?

Mobility is your access. Can your joints move through the range you need? Can your upper back rotate? Can your shoulders reach? Can your hips open? Can your ankles move? Can your spine move without one area doing everything?

After 40, many people lose range slowly. Not because their body suddenly failed. Because they stopped using certain positions. Because their habits became narrow. Because old injuries changed how they moved. Because stiffness became normal.

Mobility matters because strength needs access. If your body cannot access a position, it will either avoid it or borrow motion from somewhere else. That is where compensation begins.

The goal is not extreme flexibility. The goal is enough usable range to live, train, and move with confidence.

3. Stability: What Can You Control?

Mobility gives you access. Stability gives you ownership.

You may be able to move into a position. But can you control it? Can you balance on one leg? Can you lower into a squat without collapsing? Can you reach overhead without arching your back? Can you hinge without your low back taking over? Can you rotate without forcing? Can you breathe while holding position?

Stability is the body's confidence system. When the body does not feel stable, it often creates tension. That tension may show up as tightness, guarding, hesitation, or fear around certain movements.

This is why stability has to come before heavy intensity. Stability tells you whether your body can own the range before you ask it to load the range.

4. Strength Pattern: Who Is Doing the Work?

Strength is not only about whether you can complete the exercise. It is also about how you complete it. Who is doing the work? Where do you feel the movement? Which side dominates? What tightens first? What compensates when the movement gets hard?

This matters because your body can finish a task with the wrong strategy. A glute bridge can go to the low back. A squat can go mostly to the knees. A row can go to the neck and traps. A plank can go to the hip flexors and low back.

A strength-pattern check helps you see whether the intended areas are contributing or whether another area keeps taking over. That is how you stop building stronger compensation.

You stop asking only: Can I do it? And start asking: How is my body doing it?

5. Readiness: What Does Your Body Need Today?

Your body is not the same every day. After 40, readiness matters. Sleep matters. Stress matters. Recovery matters. Soreness matters. Pain signals matter.

This does not mean you need to overthink training. It means you need to stop ignoring context.

Some days your body is ready to train. Some days it is ready to move lightly. Some days it needs a reset. Some days it needs recovery. That is not weakness. That is wisdom.

A readiness check helps you choose the right intensity for the body you have today. Not the body you had ten years ago. Not the body you wish you had. The body in front of you.

The Structure-First Check System

Check

What It Reveals

Posture Check

Position and alignment

Mobility Check

Access and restriction

Balance Check

Control and stability

Strength Pattern Check

Weak links and compensation

Readiness Check

What your body needs today

This system is not complicated. That is the point. You do not need a hundred tests. You need a repeatable way to listen.

A few simple checks done consistently can reveal more than random workouts done aggressively. Because the checks show you where to start. And after 40, the starting point matters.

Readiness Check: Train, Reset, or Recover?

Before every workout, ask your body a few simple questions:

How is my energy today?

How did I sleep?

Am I sore or stiff?

Do I have pain that changes how I move?

Do I feel stable?

Do I feel focused?

Does my warm-up improve my movement?

Do I feel worse as I move?

This does not need to take long. You can learn a lot in three minutes.

If you feel strong, mobile, stable, and ready, train. If you feel stiff but safe, reset first and train lighter. If you feel drained, restricted, or poorly recovered, focus on reset work.

If you feel sharp pain, instability, numbness, tingling, swelling, or symptoms that concern you, stop and seek qualified guidance.

Readiness is not an excuse to avoid effort. It is a way to place effort correctly.

Assessment Gives Your Effort Direction

If you keep choosing programs that do not work, you may not have a program problem first. You may have a starting-point problem.

If the same tightness keeps returning, you may need to assess why the body keeps creating that tension.

If certain movements always feel wrong, check position, mobility, stability, and control before adding more load.

If workouts leave you beat up instead of better, you may be training harder than your structure is ready to support.

Assessment helps you stop guessing. It gives your effort direction.

How to Use Assessment Without Overthinking

Assessment should simplify training. Not complicate it. The goal is not to check everything every day. The goal is to build awareness.

Start with a few repeatable checks. Notice what keeps showing up. Use that information to choose better entry points.

If your upper body feels restricted, start with upper-chain reset work. If your low back takes over, check your core stack before loading harder. If your balance feels off, address the base before aggressive lower-body work. If your body feels beat up, reduce intensity and rebuild control.

This is not fear-based training. This is intelligent training. You are not looking for reasons to avoid work. You are looking for the right work.

The First Rule of Better Training

The first rule is not push harder. The first rule is not stretch more. The first rule is not find the perfect program.

The first rule is:

Assess before you push.

Because when you assess first, training becomes clearer. You know what needs attention. You know where to start. You know what to modify. You know when to progress. You know when to back off. You know when to seek help.

You are no longer forcing your body through someone else's map. You are learning to read your own.

That is the shift.

And once you can assess what your body is showing you, you are ready for the next step: giving your body better daily signals.

That is where the reset begins.

Part Three

The Reset

CHAPTER 8

The Daily Structure Reset

Once you can assess what your body is showing you, the next step is not to attack the body harder. The next step is to give it better signals.

That is what a reset does.

A reset is not a full workout. It is not punishment. It is not a test of toughness. It is a short, intentional sequence that helps your body find better position, better breath, better mobility, and better control before the day or before training.

After 40, this matters. Your body may not always be ready to jump straight into intensity. It may need a few minutes to shift out of stiffness. It may need to feel the ground. It may need to restore breathing. It may need to wake up the upper back. It may need to organize the ribs and pelvis. It may need to remind the hips how to move. It may need to feel safe before it produces force.

That is not weakness. That is structure.

Most people wait until their body feels bad before they give it attention. They wait until the neck is tight. Until the back is guarded. Until the hips feel locked. Until the knees complain.

A structure-first approach does not wait for the body to yell. It gives the body better input daily. Small signals. Repeated often.

Why Daily Resets Work

Your body adapts to repetition. That can work against you. It can also work for you.

If you repeat poor positions every day, the body learns them. But the same principle can be used in the other direction. If you give your body better position daily, it can learn. If you practice better breathing daily, it can learn. If you restore small ranges of motion daily, it can learn.

A daily reset works because it gives the body repeated exposure to better patterns. Not extreme patterns. Not perfect patterns. Better patterns. And better repeated long enough can become normal.

Simple Beats Complicated

A reset should be simple. If it is too complicated, you will not do it consistently. If it takes too long, you will skip it.

Five minutes done consistently can do more for awareness than a perfect routine you only do once.

The reset answers the question: What can I do today that helps my body feel more organized? That is enough.

A Reset Is Not a Cure

A daily reset is not a cure. It does not diagnose pain. It does not replace medical care. It does not solve every structural problem in five minutes.

A reset is a starting signal. It helps you notice your body. It helps you prepare your structure. It helps you reduce unnecessary tension. It helps you regain access to movement.

The reset works best when you use it as part of a larger structure-first system:

Assess → Reset → Train → Recover → Reassess

That rhythm is what changes the body over time. Not one perfect routine. A better cycle.

When To Use the Daily Reset

Use it in the morning if you wake up stiff. Use it before training if your body feels guarded. Use it after long sitting if your posture feels collapsed. Use it on low-energy days when a full workout is not realistic. Use it as a warm-up before mobility or strength work. Use it as a check-in when you are unsure what your body needs.

By the end, you should feel more aware. More upright. More grounded. More connected to your breath. More ready to move. Not destroyed. Not drained. Not sore. Ready.

The Five-Minute Daily Structure Reset

This reset has five parts:

1. Breathing Reset
2. Wall Posture Check
3. Upper-Back Opener
4. Hip Mobility Reset
5. Standing Stack Check

Move slowly. Breathe. Pay attention. If anything causes sharp pain, numbness, tingling, dizziness, or symptoms that concern you, stop and seek qualified guidance.

Step 1: Breathing Reset

Start on your back with your knees bent, or sit tall in a chair. Place one hand on your lower ribs. Place the other hand on your belly or upper chest.

Take a slow breath in through your nose if comfortable. Notice where the breath goes. Do your shoulders lift? Does your chest rise first? Do your ribs expand? Does your belly move?

Now exhale slowly. Let the ribs soften down slightly. Do not crush your abs. Do not force your ribs down. Do not hold your breath. Just exhale enough to feel the trunk settle.

Repeat for five slow breaths. The goal is not perfect breathing. The goal is awareness. You are reminding your body that the breath belongs to the structure.

What to notice: Do your shoulders relax? Does your neck soften? Does your low back feel less tense? Can you exhale without clenching?

Step 2: Wall Posture Check

Stand with your back near a wall. Place your heels a few inches away from the wall. Let your hips, upper back, and head move toward the wall naturally. Do not force the head back. Do not overarch your low back.

Can the back of your head reach the wall comfortably? Do your ribs flare to make that happen? Can you breathe in this position?

Hold for three to five slow breaths. Then step away from the wall and notice how you feel standing.

Step 3: Upper-Back Opener

Sit tall in a chair or stand with your hands lightly across your chest. Take a slow breath in. As you exhale, gently rotate your upper body to one side. Return to center. Then rotate to the other side. Move slowly. Do not twist aggressively. Keep your hips mostly facing forward. Repeat five times each side.

Then place your hands behind your head if comfortable. Gently lift your chest and upper back. Do not jam your low back. Do not crank your neck. Think of creating small movement through the upper back. Repeat five slow reps.

Step 4: Hip Mobility Reset

Stand near a wall, chair, or stable surface if needed. Place your feet about hip-width apart. Shift your hips gently side to side, then forward and back. You are waking up the hips.

Next, perform a gentle hip hinge. Place your hands on your hips. Push your hips back slightly. Keep your spine long. Let the knees bend a little. Then return to standing. Repeat five to eight reps.

Now add a small step-back reach if comfortable. Step one foot back slightly. Reach both arms forward or lightly hold support. Feel the front of the back hip open. Return to standing. Repeat three to five times each side.

Step 5: Standing Stack Check

Stand tall. Place your feet into a comfortable stance. Feel three points of contact in each foot: base of the big toe, base of the little toe, and heel.

Let your knees soften slightly. Let your ribs settle over your pelvis. Let your head float over your ribcage. Let your shoulders relax. Take three slow breaths.

Do not force perfect posture. Do not lock your knees. Do not squeeze your glutes hard. Do not pull your shoulders back aggressively. Just find a position that feels grounded, upright, and breathable.

What If You Only Have Two Minutes?

Do not skip because you cannot do all five minutes. Use a shorter version.

Take three slow breaths. Stand near a wall and notice your posture. Rotate your upper back three times each side. Hinge your hips five times. Stand tall and find your foot pressure.

That is enough to send a better signal. The goal is consistency, not perfection.

What If You Feel Worse?

A reset should not make you feel worse. It may reveal stiffness. It may reveal asymmetry. It may feel awkward. But it should not create sharp pain, dizziness, numbness, tingling, instability, or increasing discomfort.

If something feels wrong, stop. Modify the movement. Make it smaller. Slow down. Use support. Skip the movement that bothers you. And if symptoms concern you or do not settle, seek qualified guidance.

A structure-first reset should make the body feel more prepared, not more threatened.

How the Reset Changes Training

When you reset before training, you change the entry point. Instead of walking into the workout stiff, guarded, and disconnected, you give your body a chance to organize first.

You may discover that some days, after the reset, your body feels ready to train. Other days, the reset may show you that your body needs lighter work. That is useful.

Because the reset is not only preparation. It is also feedback. It helps you decide: Train. Reset more. Or recover. That is intelligent training.

The Reset Is the Beginning

The Daily Structure Reset is not the whole program. It is the beginning.

It helps you stop entering the day from stiffness. It helps you stop entering workouts from compensation. It helps you notice what your body is showing you. It gives your structure a better signal.

Breath. Position. Mobility. Control. Ground contact.

These are simple things. But simple does not mean small.

Sometimes the body does not need a more complicated answer. Sometimes it needs a better signal repeated long enough to matter.

The next chapter builds on that signal. Because once the body has a better starting point, the next question is whether it can access and control the range it needs.

That is where mobility begins.

CHAPTER 9

Mobility That Actually Transfers

Mobility is not random stretching. That needs to be clear.

Most people think mobility means getting looser. They think if a muscle feels tight, the answer is to stretch it harder, longer, or more often.

Sometimes stretching helps. But if the same tightness keeps returning, something else may be happening. Your body may not only need more range. It may need better control of the range.

That is the difference between flexibility and mobility.

Flexibility is the ability to get into a position. Mobility is the ability to access that position, control it, and use it when you move.

That distinction matters after 40. Because the goal is not to become loose. The goal is to become capable.

You do not need random range that disappears the moment you stand up. You need usable range that helps you walk, squat, hinge, reach, rotate, climb stairs, train, recover, and move through daily life with more confidence.

That is mobility that transfers.

Why Stretching Alone Often Fails

Stretching can feel good. It can reduce tension temporarily. It can help you become aware of restricted areas. It can be useful when the body simply needs more range.

But stretching alone often fails when the tightness is not just a length problem.

Sometimes the body tightens because it does not feel stable. Sometimes it tightens because a joint does not move well. Sometimes it tightens because posture, breathing, or pelvic position keeps feeding the same pattern. Sometimes it tightens because the body does not trust the range you are trying to enter.

That is why you can stretch your hips every day and still feel tight. The body does not keep range simply because you forced it once. It keeps range when it knows how to use it.

That is why mobility has to include control.

Flexibility Gives Range. Mobility Gives Ownership.

Flexibility gives you access. Mobility gives you ownership.

A flexible person may be able to enter a position passively. But that does not mean they can control it. A mobile person can access the range and use it with strength, awareness, and coordination.

This is why someone can pass a stretch test but still move poorly during training. They may have range on the floor, but lose it when standing. They may feel loose after stretching, but their body returns to the old pattern once movement begins.

The goal is movement access that carries into real life.

Can your hips open enough to squat or hinge with better control? Can your upper back rotate enough so your neck and low back do not borrow the movement? Can your ankles move enough to support stairs, squats, lunges, and walking? Can your shoulders reach without your ribs flaring?

That is mobility that matters.

Mobility and Strength Work Together

Mobility is not the opposite of strength. Mobility and strength work together.

Mobility gives the body access to better positions. Strength gives the body capacity inside those positions.

A hip that moves well but cannot stabilize may still feel unreliable. A shoulder that has range but lacks control may still feel vulnerable. A spine that can rotate but cannot control rotation may still feel unsafe.

This is why structure-first training does not separate mobility from strength forever. It uses mobility to restore access. Then it uses control and strength to keep that access useful.

Mobility After 40 Needs a Purpose

You are restoring the range your life and training actually require. That may include:

reaching overhead without neck tension

turning your upper body without your low back doing everything

hinging at the hips without back tightness

squatting to a chair with control

walking with a longer, smoother stride

going up and down stairs with more confidence

getting to the floor and back up with less fear

pressing, pulling, carrying, and training with better positions

That is practical mobility. It serves capability. It gives strength a better place to work.

The Areas That Matter Most

You do not need to mobilize everything. The big four are:

1. Upper back
2. Shoulders
3. Hips
4. Ankles

These areas influence many common movements. When they improve, many movements begin to feel different.

Upper-Back Mobility

If your upper back is stiff, your body may borrow motion from the neck or low back. That can affect overhead reaching, twisting, pressing, pulling, and even breathing.

Upper-back mobility is not about forcing your spine into extreme positions. It is about restoring small, usable movement. Can you extend without arching your low back? Can you rotate without forcing your neck? Can you breathe while moving?

The goal is not dramatic range. The goal is better access.

Shoulder Mobility

Shoulder mobility depends on more than the shoulder joint. It depends on the shoulder blade, the ribcage, the upper back, the trunk, and the breath.

That is why shoulder stretching alone does not always fix shoulder restriction. If the ribcage flares every time you reach overhead, your body may be borrowing from the low back. If the upper back does not extend or rotate well, the shoulder may not have enough room.

Good shoulder mobility allows you to reach, press, pull, carry, and move without the neck or low back taking over.

The better question is: Can I reach without compensation? That is mobility with structure.

Hip Mobility

The hips are central to lower-body movement. They affect squats, hinges, stairs, walking, lunges, rotation, posture, and low-back comfort.

When the hips are restricted, the body often borrows motion from the low back or knees. Hip mobility is not only about stretching the hip flexors. The hips need to flex, extend, rotate, and stabilize. They need access and control.

The goal is usable hip range. Enough to move, train, stand, walk, and build strength without the low back doing every job.

Ankle Mobility

Ankles are easy to ignore until they limit everything. The ankle affects squatting, stairs, walking, lunges, balance, knee tracking, and lower-body control.

If the ankle lacks mobility, the body may adjust above it. The foot may turn out. The heel may lift. The knee may cave or shift. The hip may change strategy.

You do not need extreme ankle range. You need enough motion to move through daily life and training without constant compensation.

Mobility Must Be Controlled

This is where many people miss it. They stretch. They open. They loosen. Then they walk away without teaching the body how to control the new range. The body may respond by tightening again.

Control tells the body: I can use this position.

That is why mobility work should often include slow movement, pauses, breathing, and active effort. Not aggressive force. Not bouncing. Not rushing.

Controlled mobility may look simple. A slow reach. A controlled hip shift. A gentle rotation. A squat-to-chair. These small movements teach the body to own range. That ownership is what transfers.

The Ten-Minute Mobility Reset

This reset is designed to restore access without overwhelming the body. Use it after the Daily Structure Reset, before training, after long sitting, or on days when you feel stiff.

Move slowly. Stay in a comfortable range. Do not force pain. If anything causes sharp pain, numbness, tingling, dizziness, instability, or symptoms that concern you, stop and seek qualified guidance.

Step 1: Upper-Back Rotation

Sit tall or stand with your feet grounded. Cross your arms gently over your chest. Rotate your upper body to one side. Return to center. Rotate to the other side. Move slowly. Keep your hips mostly forward. Repeat five times each side.

What to notice: Does one side feel tighter? Do you feel the movement in your upper back? Does your neck try to lead? Can you breathe while rotating?

Step 2: Shoulder Reach With Rib Control

Stand tall or sit upright. Let your ribs settle. Reach one arm overhead slowly. Do not let your ribs flare hard. Do not arch your low back to make the reach bigger. Lower the arm. Repeat on the other side. Five slow reps each side.

What to notice: Can you reach without shrugging? Does your low back arch? Do your ribs lift? Can you breathe at the top?

Step 3: Hip Shift

Stand near a wall, chair, or stable surface. Place your feet about hip-width apart. Shift your hips gently to one side. Then shift to the other side. Keep your feet grounded. Move slowly. Repeat five to eight times each side.

Step 4: Hip Hinge Reach

Stand with your feet about hip-width apart. Push your hips back. Let your knees bend slightly. Keep your spine long. Return to standing. Move slowly. Repeat six to eight reps.

What to notice: Do you feel your hips move back? Do your hamstrings load lightly? Does your low back tighten? Does your weight stay balanced through your feet?

Step 5: Ankle Rock

Stand facing a wall or chair for support. Place one foot slightly forward. Keep the heel down. Gently move the knee forward over the foot. Do not let the arch collapse. Return to start. Repeat eight to ten slow reps each side.

What to notice: Can the knee move forward without the heel lifting? Does one ankle feel more restricted? Can you keep steady pressure through the foot tripod?

Step 6: Controlled Sit-to-Stand

Stand in front of a chair. Sit back slowly until you touch the chair. Stand back up with control. Do not drop. Do not use momentum. Keep your feet grounded. Repeat five to eight reps.

What to notice: Do your knees cave inward? Does one side work harder? Does your low back take over? Can you control the lowering?

Mobility Is a Doorway

Mobility is not the destination. It is a doorway.

It opens access to better movement. It gives the body more options. It helps reduce the need for compensation. It prepares the body for strength.

But once the door opens, you still have to walk through it. That means the next layer is control. Can you own the position? Can you stabilize the range? Can you move without panic, collapse, or compensation? Can you prepare the body for load?

That is where we go next. Because before intensity, the body needs stability.

CHAPTER 10

Stability Before Intensity

Mobility opens the door. Stability teaches your body how to own what it just accessed.

That is the next layer.

Because movement without control can still feel unsafe. You may gain range, but if your body does not know how to stabilize that range, it may tighten again. It may guard. It may avoid the position. It may borrow from somewhere else.

That is why stability comes before intensity.

Not because intensity is bad. Intensity matters. Strength matters. Load matters. Challenge matters.

But if you add intensity to a pattern your body does not control, the body will usually find a workaround. The knee caves. The low back arches. The shoulder shrugs. The neck tightens. The feet collapse. The hips shift. The breath disappears.

You may still complete the exercise. But completion is not the same as control. And after 40, that difference matters.

At DominionBuilt, the rule is simple:

Control comes before load.

Before you ask your body to lift more, push harder, or move faster, you need to know whether it can control the position, the range, and the pattern.

That is what stability gives you.

Stability Is Not Stiffness

Many people confuse stability with stiffness. They think being stable means locking everything down. Tight abs. Rigid posture. Hard bracing. No movement.

But real stability is not stiffness. Stability is controlled freedom.

It is the ability to move without collapsing. To hold position without gripping. To resist unwanted movement without becoming rigid. To breathe while under effort. To stay organized when the exercise gets harder.

Real stability gives the body confidence. It lets your joints move with support. It helps you feel safer in positions that used to feel uncertain. It gives strength somewhere to land.

Why Instability Feels Like Weakness

Sometimes what you call weakness is really instability.

You may think your legs are weak because lunges feel shaky. But the issue may be balance, hip control, foot pressure, or trunk stability.

You may think your shoulders are weak because pressing feels awkward. But the issue may be shoulder blade control, rib position, upper-back movement, or poor trunk support.

You may think your core is weak because planks feel hard. But the issue may be breathing, bracing, rib flare, pelvic position, or low-back compensation.

Weakness may be part of the picture. But instability often makes weakness feel worse.

Stability gives the body better tools.

The Body Protects What It Does Not Trust

Your body does not like uncertainty. If a joint feels unsupported, the body may guard it. If a range feels unfamiliar, the body may avoid it. If a movement feels uncontrolled, the body may reduce power.

This is protection. And protection is not always wrong. If something is truly unsafe, the body should protect you. The problem is when protection becomes the default.

A body that constantly protects itself can start to feel stiff, weak, hesitant, and unreliable. You may feel like you have to warm up forever. You may avoid deeper positions. You may feel nervous under load. You may stop trusting certain movements.

Stability helps restore trust. Not by forcing the body. But by proving, through repeated controlled movement, that the position can be owned.

Stability Lives in the Whole System

Stability is not only a core issue. It lives through the whole body.

Your feet help stabilize your base. Your hips help stabilize your pelvis and lower body. Your trunk helps stabilize the spine and transfer force. Your shoulder blades help stabilize the upper body. Your breath helps organize pressure and control.

That is why one unstable area can affect the entire movement. If the feet are unstable, the knees and hips may adjust. If the hips are unstable, the trunk may compensate. If the trunk is unstable, the shoulders and low back may work harder.

The body does not isolate stability. It shares it. That is why the structure-first sequence matters:

Position → Control → Load → Capacity

Tempo Reveals Control

One of the simplest ways to build stability is to slow down.

Speed can hide problems. Momentum can help you escape weak positions. Fast reps can let you bounce through ranges you do not actually own. But tempo reveals truth.

When you slow a movement down, you can feel where the body shifts, where tension appears, where balance changes, where control disappears, whether you can breathe.

A slow squat-to-chair reveals the base. A slow hinge reveals the hips and trunk. A slow wall push-up reveals shoulder and core control. A slow step-down reveals hip, knee, ankle, and foot coordination.

Slow does not mean easy. Slow often makes the movement more honest. And after 40, honest movement is valuable.

Balance Is Stability in Motion

Balance is not separate from stability. Balance is stability in motion.

When you stand on one leg, step down, lunge, walk on uneven ground, or carry something heavy, your body has to organize quickly. Your foot has to connect. Your ankle has to respond. Your knee has to track. Your hip has to stabilize. Your trunk has to stay organized. Your breathing has to continue.

You need to step off a curb without panic. You need to go downstairs with confidence. You need to carry groceries without feeling unstable. You need to move through life without every small shift feeling risky.

Balance is not only about preventing falls. It is about restoring confidence in movement.

Stability Before Load

Load exposes structure. If the pattern is controlled, load can build strength. If the pattern is unstable, load may expose compensation.

A body that can control a squat-to-chair is better prepared to squat with weight. A body that can hinge without the low back taking over is better prepared to deadlift. A body that can reach overhead without rib flare or neck tension is better prepared to press. A body that can brace and breathe is better prepared to carry, pull, push, and train with intensity.

This is the difference between training hard and training recklessly.

Training hard respects the body's current capacity. Training recklessly ignores it.

The goal is not to stay in beginner mode forever. The goal is to build the right to progress.

The Foundation Stability Circuit

This circuit is not designed to exhaust you. It is designed to teach control.

Use it after the Daily Structure Reset or after mobility work. Use it before strength training. Use it on days when your body feels unstable, disconnected, or unsure.

Move slowly. Breathe. Stay in a range you can control. If anything causes sharp pain, numbness, tingling, dizziness, instability, or symptoms that concern you, stop and seek qualified guidance.

The circuit includes:

1. Dead Bug Variation
2. Bird Dog Variation
3. Glute Bridge
4. Split-Stance Hold
5. Controlled Step-Back Pattern

Movement 1: Dead Bug Variation

Lie on your back with your knees bent. Bring your legs up one at a time so your knees are over your hips if comfortable. Reach your arms toward the ceiling.

Let your ribs settle. Keep your low back from arching hard. Take a slow breath in. As you exhale, slowly lower one heel toward the floor. Bring it back. Alternate sides. Keep the movement small if needed.

What to notice: Do your ribs flare? Does your low back arch? Do your hip flexors grip? Can you move slowly? Can you breathe?

Start with 5 slow reps per side. Stop before your low back takes over.

Movement 2: Bird Dog Variation

Start on hands and knees. Place your hands under your shoulders. Place your knees under your hips. Find a long spine.

Reach one leg back slowly. If that feels controlled, reach the opposite arm forward. Pause briefly. Return to the starting position. Alternate sides. Keep the movement slow and controlled.

What to notice: Does your body shift side to side? Does your low back arch? Do your hips rotate? Can you keep your neck relaxed? Can you breathe?

Start with 4–6 slow reps per side.

Movement 3: Glute Bridge

Lie on your back with your knees bent and feet on the floor. Place your feet about hip-width apart. Let your ribs settle. Gently press through your feet. Lift your hips until your body forms a straight line from shoulders to knees.

Do not overarch your low back. Do not flare your ribs. Pause briefly at the top. Lower with control.

What to notice: Do you feel glutes or mostly low back? Do your hamstrings cramp? Do your ribs flare? Do your knees drift out or cave in?

Start with 8 slow reps. Focus on control, not height.

Movement 4: Split-Stance Hold

Stand near a wall or chair for support. Step one foot back slightly so you are in a split stance. Both feet stay grounded. Keep your front foot steady. Let your knees soften. Stack your ribs over your pelvis. Breathe. Hold the position. Switch sides.

What to notice: Does one side feel less stable? Does your front foot grip the floor? Does your knee wobble? Does your hip shift?

Start with 15–20 seconds per side. Use support as needed.

Movement 5: Controlled Step-Back Pattern

Stand tall with feet grounded. Shift weight onto one foot. Slowly step the other foot back. Touch the toes lightly to the floor. Return to standing. Alternate sides or complete one side at a time. Use a wall or chair for support if needed. Move slowly.

What to notice: Does your front knee cave? Does your foot collapse? Does your hip shift? Do you lose balance? Does your trunk lean heavily?

Start with 5 slow reps per side. Stay within a range you can control.

How to Use the Circuit

Start with one round. If your body feels good, repeat for a second round. Do not chase fatigue. Chase quality.

Movement

Starting Amount

Dead Bug Variation

5 reps per side

Bird Dog Variation

4–6 reps per side

Glute Bridge

8 reps

Split-Stance Hold

15–20 seconds per side

Controlled Step-Back

5 reps per side

Move slowly. Rest as needed. Breathe. The circuit should leave you feeling more connected, not crushed. If your form gets worse, stop there. That is the signal.

What If Stability Work Feels Too Easy?

Stability work can look easy. That does not mean it is useless. The question is not whether the movement looks hard. The question is whether you can control it well.

Can you breathe? Can you keep position? Can you move slowly? Can you avoid compensation? Can you feel the right areas working?

If the answer is yes, then you can progress. Progress may mean slowing the movement down, adding a pause, increasing range slightly, reducing support, adding light resistance, or moving to a harder variation.

But progress should not destroy control. If the pattern breaks, the load or difficulty is too high for now.

What If Stability Work Feels Hard?

If stability work feels harder than expected, pay attention. That may explain why heavier training has felt frustrating. Your body may be telling you that control is the missing layer.

Make the movement smaller. Use support. Reduce reps. Slow down. Choose the easier version.

Many people want to rush past this work because it does not feel exciting. But the body often needs these basics more than another intense workout.

Simple done well can rebuild trust.

How Stability Changes Strength Training

When stability improves, strength training usually feels different. You may feel more grounded during lower-body work. You may feel less low-back takeover. You may feel your glutes contribute better. You may control your knees more easily. You may press or pull with less neck tension. You may balance better. You may recover with less guarding.

That is not because stability replaces strength. It prepares the body to express strength better.

This is why stability belongs before intensity. Not instead of intensity. Before intensity.

Once the body controls the pattern, load becomes more useful.

Stability Is the Final Gate Before Strength

You have now seen the sequence.

First, assess. Then reset. Then restore mobility that transfers. Then build stability.

This is the final gate before strength.

Not because strength is dangerous. Strength is necessary. But strength works best when the body has a foundation it can trust.

You do not need to be perfect before you train. You do not need flawless movement. You do not need endless corrective exercises.

But you do need enough position, mobility, and stability to make strength productive.

That is where the next chapter begins. Because after 40, strength still matters. It may matter more than ever.

But it must be built with better rules.

CHAPTER 11

Strength After 40: Build Without Breaking Down

The most common mistake in strength training after 40 is not training too little. It is training without changing the entry point when the body shows compensation. Someone adds weight to a press they have been doing for months. The shoulder starts to ache. The instinct is to push through or drop the weight. The better question is: where is the ribcage during the press? Where are the shoulder blades? Changing the entry point — starting from a better position, with less range until control returns — often fixes the complaint without changing the exercise.

Strength still matters after 40.

In many ways, it matters more.

Strength helps you move with confidence. It helps you protect your independence. It helps you carry, climb, lift, stand, walk, train, and live with more capacity. It helps your body hold onto muscle. It helps your joints feel more supported. It helps your posture have something behind it. It helps your body feel capable again.

But strength after 40 needs better rules.

Not fearful rules. Not weak rules. Smarter rules.

Because the goal is not just to work hard. The goal is to build strength your body can keep.

A younger body may tolerate sloppy training longer. It may recover faster from poor decisions. It may absorb random programming for a season.

But after 40, the body usually becomes more honest. It tells you when the warm-up was not enough. It tells you when the load was too heavy too soon. It tells you when your mobility was not ready. It tells you when your low back did too much. It tells you when your knees were not tracking well. It tells you when your shoulders were not supported.

That is not betrayal. That is feedback.

Strength after 40 is not about proving you are still young. It is about building a body that is strong, prepared, controlled, and resilient in the stage you are actually in.

At DominionBuilt, the goal is simple:

Build strength without breaking down.

Strength Is Not the Problem

Strength training is not the enemy. Aging is not a reason to avoid resistance.

Your body still needs challenge. Your muscles still need tension. Your bones still need load. Your joints still need movement. Your nervous system still needs practice. Your body still needs to be reminded that it is capable.

The problem is not strength. The problem is strength built without structure.

It is loading poor positions. It is rushing progression. It is chasing soreness. It is copying workouts that do not fit your body. It is adding intensity before control. It is ignoring readiness. It is treating every training day like your body is the same.

They do not fail because strength training is bad. They struggle because the strength work is not matched to the body in front of them.

A structure-first approach does not tell you to stop getting strong. It teaches you how to earn strength again.

The New Rule: Productive Challenge

After 40, not every hard workout is a good workout.

Hard is not enough. Sweat is not enough. Soreness is not proof. Exhaustion is not the goal.

The better question is: Was the challenge productive?

A productive challenge builds capacity without creating unnecessary breakdown. It asks enough from the body to create adaptation. But not so much that the body leaves the session more guarded, irritated, or unstable than before.

A productive challenge should make you feel like you trained. But it should not make you feel punished. It should expose weak links. But it should not recklessly overload them. It should build confidence. Not make you fear the next session.

The goal is not easy training. The goal is useful training. There is a difference.

Strength Needs the Right Entry Point

Every exercise has an entry point. The entry point is the version your body can perform with good enough position, control, and confidence today.

Not the version your ego wants. Not the version you used to do. Not the version someone online is doing. The version your body can own now.

A squat may begin with a squat-to-chair. A deadlift may begin with a hip hinge drill. A lunge may begin with a split-stance hold. A push-up may begin at a wall or elevated surface. An overhead press may begin with a landmine press, incline press, or controlled shoulder reach. A loaded carry may begin with a light suitcase carry.

That is not regression. That is strategy.

The wrong entry point can make a good exercise feel bad. The right entry point can make a difficult pattern trainable again.

You do not force your body into the hardest version first. You choose the version that teaches the body how to succeed.

Do Not Confuse Modification With Weakness

Modification is not weakness. Modification is precision.

A person with wisdom modifies the exercise to match the structure. A person with ego forces the body into a version it does not control.

That does not mean you stay modified forever. It means you build from the correct step.

If the knees cave during lunges, you may need a supported split squat first. If the low back takes over during deadlifts, you may need hinge patterning before loading heavy. If push-ups irritate the shoulders, you may need elevated push-ups, better scapular control, or a different pressing angle. If overhead pressing creates neck tension, you may need upper-chain and core-stack work before heavy overhead load.

The goal is not to avoid hard things. The goal is to make hard things build you instead of break you.

Modification gives the body a better path. And a better path repeated consistently becomes progress.

The Five Strength Patterns That Matter

You do not need endless exercises. You need to build the major patterns well.

For most adults over 40, the key strength patterns are:

Squat

Hinge

Push

Pull

Carry

These patterns cover a lot of life.

Squat helps you sit, stand, climb, and lower. Hinge helps you bend, lift, reach, and protect your back. Push helps you press, rise, brace, and move things away from you. Pull helps your posture, upper back, shoulders, and daily lifting. Carry helps your grip, trunk, posture, balance, and total-body strength.

You can build a strong body with these patterns. But each pattern has to be matched to your current structure.

The question is not: What is the hardest version I can survive?

The better question is: What is the cleanest version I can build from?

That question keeps strength productive.

Pattern 1: Squat

The squat pattern matters because you use it every day. Every time you sit down, stand up, lower yourself, climb stairs, or pick something up from a low position, some version of the squat is involved.

But not every body needs the same squat. Some people can squat deeply with control. Some need a chair. Some need a box. Some need a wider stance. Some need heel elevation. Some need better ankle mobility. Some need more hip control. Some need to slow down and rebuild the pattern.

A structure-first squat asks: Can the feet stay grounded? Can the knees track with control? Can the hips contribute? Can the trunk stay organized? Can the movement be lowered with control? Can the person stand without momentum?

If the answer is no, the squat needs an easier entry point. That may mean using a chair, reducing depth, holding support, slowing the tempo, lightening the load, or improving mobility and stability first.

The squat is not just a leg exercise. It is a full structure check.

Pattern 2: Hinge

The hinge is one of the most important patterns to rebuild after 40. It teaches the hips to move while the spine stays organized.

This matters for deadlifts. But it also matters for daily life. Picking something up. Loading groceries. Leaning over a sink. Reaching into a trunk. Lifting a laundry basket. Working in the yard. Playing with children or grandchildren.

The hinge protects your back by teaching your hips to do their job.

But many people do not hinge well. They round through the spine. They squat instead of hinging. They arch the low back. They shift to one side. They feel everything in the back and nothing in the hips.

Before loading a hinge heavily, the body should learn: hips move back, spine stays long, ribs stay controlled, feet stay grounded, hamstrings load, low back does not dominate, breath stays steady.

A hinge does not need to be heavy to be valuable. A clean hinge is a foundation. Once that foundation is built, load can become useful.

Pattern 3: Push

The push pattern includes movements like push-ups, chest presses, overhead presses, and pressing objects away from the body. Pushing helps build the chest, shoulders, triceps, and trunk.

But after 40, pushing often reveals upper-chain issues. The shoulders may roll forward. The neck may tighten. The low back may arch. The ribs may flare. The shoulder blades may not move well.

This is why pressing must be chosen carefully. A person who struggles with floor push-ups may do better with wall push-ups or elevated push-ups. A person who arches during overhead pressing may need a different angle first. A person with shoulder irritation may need to improve pulling strength, upper-back mobility, and shoulder blade control.

The push pattern should not feel like the neck is doing the work. It should not feel like the low back is helping press the weight. It should not feel unstable through the shoulder.

The question is: Can I push while staying organized? If yes, progress. If not, change the entry point.

Pattern 4: Pull

Pulling is one of the most important patterns for adults over 40. It supports the upper back. It helps balance the shoulders. It reinforces posture. It trains the back, arms, grip, and trunk. It helps counter some of the forward-dominant positions of modern life.

Rows, pulldowns, assisted pulls, cable pulls, band pulls, and carries can all support this pattern.

But pulling also has to be done with control. Many people turn rows into shrugging. They feel traps and neck more than mid-back. They yank the weight. They overarch the low back. They pull with the arms but never organize the shoulder blades.

A structure-first pull asks: Can the neck stay relaxed? Can the shoulder blades move without shrugging? Can the ribs stay controlled? Can the trunk stay steady? Can the back contribute without yanking? Can the movement be lowered slowly?

Pulling should help restore the upper chain. Not feed more tension into it. When pulling is done well, it can become one of the strongest tools for posture, shoulder support, and upper-body strength.

Pattern 5: Carry

Carries are simple. That is why they are powerful.

Pick something up. Hold it. Walk with control.

A carry trains grip, shoulders, trunk, hips, feet, posture, breathing, and balance at the same time. It is strength you can feel in real life.

Carrying groceries. Holding bags. Moving furniture. Carrying a child. Walking with load. Staying upright under weight.

Carries teach the body to organize under demand. But even carries need the right entry point.

Start light. Stand tall. Keep the ribs and pelvis organized. Do not lean hard to one side. Do not let the shoulders shrug. Do not hold your breath. Keep the steps controlled.

A suitcase carry, where weight is held on one side, can teach trunk control. A farmer's carry, with weight in both hands, can build total-body strength. A front carry can teach bracing.

The goal is not to see how much you can suffer through. The goal is to carry with structure.

How Heavy Should You Go?

Heavy is relative. A weight that is light for one person may be heavy for another. A weight that was easy ten years ago may not be the right starting point today.

The better question is not only: Can I lift it? The better question is: Can I control it?

Use these questions: Can I keep position? Can I move through the range without pain? Can I breathe? Can I control the lowering? Can I avoid compensating? Can I repeat the rep cleanly? Can I recover from the session?

If the answer is yes, the weight may be appropriate. If the answer is no, the weight is too heavy for that pattern right now.

Not too heavy for your worth. Too heavy for your current structure. That distinction matters.

Leave Reps in Reserve

After 40, you do not need every set to be a battle. You do not need to train to failure on every exercise. You do not need to turn every workout into a test.

A better rule is to leave reps in reserve. That means you stop the set before your form falls apart. You finish knowing you could have done a little more with good control.

This helps you build strength without constantly draining recovery. For many adults over 40, leaving one to three good reps in reserve is often a smarter default than grinding every set to failure.

That does not mean you never work hard. It means your hard work is governed. Your body should leave the session with a signal to adapt. Not a demand to survive.

That is how you build consistency.

Progress Slowly Enough To Keep Winning

Progress matters. You should get stronger. But progress does not only mean adding weight.

Progress can mean:

better control

more range

smoother reps

less compensation

better balance

better breathing

more confidence

more reps with the same weight

more sets with clean form

slower tempo

shorter rest

slightly heavier load

This matters because many people only respect one kind of progress: more weight. But if you add weight while losing control, that is not true progress. That may be compensation dressed up as strength.

A structure-first body progresses in layers. First, own the pattern. Then repeat it. Then add capacity. Then add load. Then build intensity.

This keeps the body moving forward without constantly resetting from flare-ups.

Soreness Is Not the Scorecard

Soreness is not the goal. You may get sore sometimes. That is normal. But soreness does not prove the workout was effective. And lack of soreness does not prove the workout failed.

After 40, chasing soreness can become expensive. It can disrupt recovery. It can affect the next workout. It can make joints feel guarded. It can make movement feel worse.

A better scorecard is: Did I move better? Did I train the intended pattern? Did I keep control? Did I challenge myself appropriately? Did I leave with more confidence? Can I recover and repeat the work?

The goal is not to limp away from training. The goal is to build capacity.

Capacity means your body can do more, tolerate more, recover better, and keep showing up. That is stronger than soreness.

Recovery Is Part of Strength

Strength is not built only during the workout. The workout gives the signal. Recovery allows the body to adapt. If recovery is poor, progress slows.

If stress is high, recovery changes. If sleep is poor, recovery changes. If nutrition is inconsistent, recovery changes. If you train hard every day with no respect for readiness, recovery changes.

This matters more after 40. You can still train hard. But you need to recover intentionally.

That may mean spacing hard sessions better. Alternating heavy and lighter days. Using reset work between training days. Walking. Sleeping better. Managing stress. Eating enough protein. Listening when the body feels unusually guarded.

Recovery is not laziness. Recovery is part of the system. A body that recovers well can train more consistently. A body that never recovers eventually pushes back.

The Strength Session Should Have Order

A good strength session does not need to be complicated. But it should have order.

A simple structure may look like this:

Assess — Notice readiness, stiffness, pain, and control

Reset — Give the body better signals before movement

Prepare the pattern — Practice the movement before load

Train the main strength movement — Build capacity

Add support work — Address weak links

Cool down or recover — Help the body come down from the session

This is not fancy. It is organized. And organized training beats random intensity.

WHAT THIS EXPLAINS

If lifting leaves you feeling beat up, the issue may not be strength training itself. It may be the entry point, load, exercise selection, readiness, or recovery.

If you always feel the wrong muscles working, your body may need better structure before heavier loading.

If your low back takes over during lower-body training, your hinge, squat, core stack, or hip control may need attention.

If your neck tightens during upper-body training, your upper chain, shoulder blade control, rib position, or breathing may be part of the pattern.

If you cannot stay consistent, the workouts may be costing more than your body can recover from.

If you feel like you have to start over again and again, you may be progressing load faster than you are progressing control.

Strength after 40 is not about doing less. It is about building better.

The Goal Is Capacity

The goal is not one impressive workout. The goal is capacity.

Capacity means you can do more over time. Move better. Train consistently. Recover well. Build strength. Handle daily life. Trust your body. Stay active. Return to movement when life interrupts. Progress without constantly feeling like you are one mistake away from pain.

That is what strength should give you. Not just bigger numbers. More capability. More confidence. More freedom.

A strong body after 40 is not a body that ignores signals. It is a body that reads them, responds wisely, and keeps building.

That is the DominionBuilt way.

Build Strength Your Body Can Keep

You do not need to prove anything to your younger self. You do not need to punish your body into progress. You do not need to chase the hardest version of every exercise.

You need to build strength your body can keep.

That means choosing the right entry point. Respecting position. Owning control. Using load wisely. Progressing with patience. Recovering with intention. And training in a way that lets you come back again.

Strength is still available. Progress is still available. Capacity is still available.

But the rules have changed.

Not because your body is broken. Because your body is asking for better structure.

And when strength is built on structure, it can become one of the greatest tools you have for the years ahead.

CHAPTER 12

Recovery Is Training

Most people think recovery means doing nothing.

They think training is the work. Recovery is the break. Training is discipline. Recovery is rest. Training builds the body. Recovery is what happens when you cannot train.

But that is not the full truth.

Recovery is not separate from training. Recovery is part of training.

The workout gives the body a signal. Recovery is where the body responds. Recovery is the process that allows your body to absorb training, repair, adapt, and return ready for the next signal.

If the signal is good but recovery is poor, progress suffers. If the workout is hard but the body never gets enough time, sleep, nutrition, or downshift to adapt, training starts to feel like breakdown.

That is why recovery matters more after 40. Not because you are weak. Because your body is more honest now.

It may not tolerate poor sleep, high stress, random workouts, and aggressive intensity the same way it once did. It may tell you sooner. Through stiffness.

Through soreness that lingers. Through joints that feel irritated. Through workouts that feel harder than they should. Through motivation that drops. Through strength that does not move. Through a body that feels guarded before you even begin.

That is not failure. That is feedback.

At DominionBuilt, the principle is simple:

Recovery is training.

Because a body that cannot recover cannot keep building.

The Workout Is Only the Signal

Training does not make you stronger by itself. Training challenges the body. It creates a demand. It tells the body: Adapt to this.

But the adaptation does not fully happen during the workout. It happens after. When you sleep. When you eat. When you hydrate. When your nervous system calms down. When tissues repair. When the body has time to rebuild.

That is why harder is not always better. If the workout signal is too much for your recovery capacity, the body may not adapt well. It may protect. It may tighten. It may feel drained. It may reduce output. It may make the next workout worse.

A good training plan does not only ask: Can I survive this workout? It asks: Can I recover from this workout and come back better?

That question changes everything.

After 40, Recovery Becomes More Valuable

A younger body may cover a lot of mistakes. Poor warm-ups. Bad sleep. Random meals. Hard training stacked too close together. Too much volume. Too much intensity. Too little mobility. Too little recovery.

But after 40, the margin often gets smaller.

You can still train hard. You can still get stronger. You can still build muscle. You can still improve mobility, stability, posture, and capacity. But recovery has to be respected.

Your body may need more preparation. More intentional progression. More attention to sleep. More attention to stress. More attention to what happens between workouts.

This is not a downgrade. It is refinement. You are no longer training from assumption. You are training from wisdom.

Stress Counts as Load

Your body does not only respond to gym stress. It responds to life stress.

Work stress. Family stress. Financial stress. Emotional stress. Poor sleep. Long sitting. Travel. Conflict. Mental overload. A full schedule.

Your body has to recover from all of it. That means stress counts as load.

You may not be holding a dumbbell. But your system is still carrying weight.

This matters because people often judge their training capacity only by the workout. They say: It was only thirty minutes. It was not that heavy. But the body is not only responding to the workout. It is responding to the full load of your life.

If life stress is high, training may need to be adjusted. Not abandoned. Adjusted. That is not weakness. That is intelligent programming.

When Recovery Is Poor, Compensation Increases

A tired body compensates faster. When recovery is poor, control drops. Balance changes. Coordination changes. Bracing changes. Mobility may feel worse. The body may guard more.

The low back may take over. The knees may feel less supported. The neck and shoulders may tighten. Movements that usually feel fine may suddenly feel off.

That does not always mean the exercise became bad. It may mean your system was not ready.

This is why readiness matters. A poorly recovered body may still be able to train. But it may need a different kind of session. Less load. Less volume. More reset work. More walking. More mobility. More stability. More technique.

The goal is not to quit every time you feel tired. The goal is to choose the kind of work your body can actually use.

Sleep Is the Foundation

Sleep is one of the most important recovery tools you have.

It affects energy, mood, pain sensitivity, strength, coordination, decision-making, motivation, and recovery.

A poor night of sleep does not mean the day is ruined. But if poor sleep becomes the pattern, training will usually feel different. You may feel more stiff, more irritable, less coordinated, less strong, less motivated, more sensitive to discomfort, and more likely to compensate.

This is why sleep matters for structure-first training. A body that does not sleep well often struggles to recover well. And a body that does not recover well has a harder time building strength.

You do not need perfect sleep. But you do need to respect sleep as part of the system.

Better sleep is not just a lifestyle tip. It is training support.

Food Supports Recovery

This is not a diet book. But recovery still needs fuel.

Your body needs enough protein to support muscle repair. Enough calories to support training. Enough fluids to support function. Enough nutrients to support energy, tissue health, and daily movement.

If you under-eat while training hard, recovery may suffer. If you skip protein repeatedly, rebuilding becomes harder. If you live dehydrated, your body may feel worse than it needs to.

This does not mean you need a perfect meal plan. It means your body needs materials to rebuild. Training asks the body to adapt. Food helps provide the resources.

You cannot build well without giving the body something to build with.

Walking Helps Recovery

Walking is one of the most underrated recovery tools.

It is simple. It is accessible for many people. It helps circulation. It supports joint motion. It reinforces gait. It can reduce stiffness. It can calm the nervous system. It can help digestion. It can give the body movement without heavy stress.

Walking is not just cardio. It is low-level structure work. Every step gives your feet, ankles, knees, hips, trunk, shoulders, and arms a chance to coordinate.

A relaxed walk can help the body downshift from harder training. It can also keep you moving on days when a full workout is not the right choice.

You do not need to turn every walk into a performance. Sometimes the value is in the rhythm. Move. Breathe. Let the body cycle. That is recovery.

Reset Days Are Not Wasted Days

A reset day is not a failed workout day. It is a training day with a different purpose.

Some days, your body does not need more intensity. It needs better signals. Breathing. Mobility. Stability. Light movement. Walking. Gentle pattern practice.

A reset day can help you maintain rhythm without forcing load. This is important for consistency.

Many people think they only have two options: train hard or do nothing. That mindset creates problems. Because when the body is not ready for hard training, they either push through and feel worse, or they stop completely and lose rhythm.

A reset day gives you a third option. You still show up. You still move. You still support the body. But you do it in a way your system can receive.

That is how consistency survives real life.

The Recovery Check

Before you train, ask a few recovery questions:

How did I sleep?

How is my energy?

Am I still sore from the last workout?

Do my joints feel irritated?

Do I feel more stiff than usual?

Is my stress high today?

Does my warm-up make me feel better or worse?

Do I feel focused and coordinated?

Can I breathe well during movement?

Do I feel ready to add load?

You are looking for direction. If most answers are positive, train. If answers are mixed, train lighter or reduce volume. If answers are poor, reset and recover. If there are concerning symptoms, stop and seek qualified guidance.

This is not about fear. It is about matching the day's work to the body's readiness.

Train, Reset, or Recover

The goal is not to make every day the same. The goal is to make every day useful.

A train day means the body is ready for productive challenge. You can load. You can progress. You can build.

A reset day means the body needs movement, but not heavy stress. You focus on breath, mobility, stability, walking, and light pattern work.

A recovery day means the body needs restoration. You may walk lightly, rest, sleep, hydrate, eat well, and let the body adapt.

Here is a simple rule: If movement improves as you warm up, train or train lighter. If movement gets worse as you warm up, reset or recover.

That rule will not answer everything. But it gives you a better starting point than ignoring the signal.

Each day has value. The mature athlete understands the difference. The wise adult learns the rhythm.

Signs You May Need More Recovery

Your body usually gives signs. You may need more recovery if:

soreness lasts longer than usual

joints feel irritated

motivation drops sharply

sleep gets worse

strength drops for multiple sessions

movements feel less coordinated

stiffness increases instead of improving

the same areas keep tightening

your resting energy feels low

every workout feels harder than it should

you feel more guarded after training than before

These signs do not mean panic. They mean pay attention. Sometimes the answer is simple. Reduce volume. Take a lighter day. Walk. Sleep. Eat better. Reset. Give your body time.

Recovery is not quitting. Recovery is how you keep building.

Recovery and Pain Signals

Pain changes the conversation.

This book is not a medical guide. If you have sharp pain, numbness, tingling, swelling, sudden weakness, trauma, chest pain, dizziness, unexplained symptoms, or pain that does not settle, seek qualified care. Do not try to prove toughness through warning signs. That is not wisdom.

But not every sensation is an emergency. Some discomfort may be muscular. Some stiffness may improve with movement. Some soreness may be normal after training.

The key is to observe. Does movement make it better or worse? Does the sensation change your mechanics? Does it increase as you continue? Does it linger longer than expected? Does it feel sharp, unstable, or concerning?

A structure-first body listens early. It does not ignore signals until they become louder.

How Recovery Changes Strength

When recovery improves, strength often improves. Not because you suddenly became more disciplined. Because your body finally has room to adapt.

You may notice: better energy, better mobility, better coordination, stronger lifts, less joint irritation, better mood, better consistency, less fear around training, fewer setbacks, more confidence.

That is the fruit of recovery.

Training gives the signal. Recovery lets the signal become progress. If you only chase the signal and ignore the adaptation, you stay stuck in stress. But when you respect both, training becomes sustainable.

WHAT THIS EXPLAINS

If you train hard but feel worse over time, recovery may be the missing piece.

If you keep getting tight in the same places, your body may not be recovering enough to release guarding.

If your strength fluctuates wildly, sleep, stress, food, and readiness may be affecting your output.

If mobility feels better one day and worse the next, recovery and nervous system state may be part of the pattern.

If you cannot stay consistent, your plan may not include enough reset and recovery options.

If you feel guilty on lighter days, you may be confusing exhaustion with progress.

Recovery helps you stop fighting the body. It teaches you how to work with it.

Recovery Is a Skill

Recovery is not just something that happens. It is something you practice.

You practice ending a workout before form falls apart. You practice sleeping with more intention. You practice walking instead of doing nothing. You practice taking lighter days without guilt. You practice eating enough to support training. You practice reducing stress when possible. You practice listening before the body has to yell.

That is maturity. That is structure. That is how adults build strength that lasts.

Not by ignoring recovery. By training it.

Build the Body That Can Come Back

The strongest body is not the body that survives one hard session. It is the body that can come back.

Again and again. With less fear. With better control. With more capacity. With more trust.

That is the goal. Recovery is what makes that possible. It lets the body absorb the work. It lets the structure adapt. It lets strength become sustainable. It lets training become something you can keep doing.

Not for a few weeks. Not for one challenge. For the life you are still building.

Your body is not asking you to stop. It is asking you to respect the full cycle.

Assess. Reset. Train. Recover. Reassess.

Build. Reset. Recover. Repeat.

That is how the body rebuilds.

And once recovery becomes part of the system, the next step is learning how to organize the whole week. Because a strong body after 40 does not need random effort.

It needs a repeatable rhythm.

CHAPTER 13

The Weekly Rhythm: Build, Reset, Recover

A strong body after 40 does not need random effort.

It needs a repeatable rhythm.

That rhythm does not have to be complicated. It does not need to take over your life. It does not need to look like a professional athlete's schedule. It needs to make sense for the body you have, the life you live, and the capacity you are trying to rebuild.

Most people think the main question is: How many days should I work out?

That question matters. But it is not the first question.

The better question is: What rhythm can my body recover from, repeat, and build on?

Because the best program is not the one that looks impressive on paper. The best program is the one your body can actually use.

If the week is too easy, nothing changes. If the week is too aggressive, the body starts pushing back. If the week is too random, you never build momentum. If the week has no reset or recovery, training becomes a cycle of forcing and restarting.

The goal is not to punish the body into progress. The goal is to build a rhythm that keeps moving forward.

At DominionBuilt, the weekly rhythm is simple:

Build. Reset. Recover. Repeat.

Strength builds capacity. Reset restores structure. Recovery allows adaptation. Repetition turns the system into a life.

Why Random Weeks Create Random Results

Many people do not fail because they lack effort. They fail because their effort has no rhythm.

One week they train hard five days in a row. The next week they miss everything. Then they return with guilt and overdo it. Then they get sore, stiff, or irritated. Then they rest too long. Then they start over.

This cycle is common. Not because people are lazy. Because their plan does not match real life.

A random week usually has no structure. No recovery plan. No lighter option. No reset day. No rule for when the body feels off. No clear way to restart after interruption.

That makes consistency fragile.

After 40, consistency needs more than motivation. It needs a system that can bend without breaking.

A weekly rhythm gives you that. It gives you a plan for strong days. A plan for stiff days. A plan for tired days.

A plan for busy days. A plan for getting back on track without turning every missed workout into failure.

That is how you stop starting over.

The Three Types of Training Days

A structure-first week should include three types of days:

Build Days

Reset Days

Recovery Days

Each day has a different purpose.

A build day is for strength, capacity, and productive challenge. A reset day is for breath, mobility, stability, and movement quality. A recovery day is for adaptation, restoration, walking, and lower stress.

All three matter. If you only build, the body may not recover. If you only reset, the body may not get strong enough. If you only recover, the body may lose capacity.

The rhythm works because the days support each other. Build days create the signal. Reset days clean up the pattern. Recovery days let the body absorb the work. Together, they create progress you can repeat.

Build Days

Build days are the days you train strength. These are the sessions where you challenge the body with resistance, effort, and progression. But even build days should still be structure-first.

You begin with assessment. You use a reset. You prepare the pattern. Then you train.

A build day may include:

a quick readiness check

the Daily Structure Reset

mobility or stability prep

one or two main strength patterns

one or two support patterns

a recovery finish

The goal is productive challenge. Not punishment.

A good build day should leave the body feeling trained, not wrecked. You may be tired. You may feel worked. You may feel challenged. But you should not feel like your joints were punished, your low back carried the whole session, or your body was forced through patterns it did not control.

Build days should make the body more capable over time. If they keep making you feel less capable, something in the structure needs to change.

Reset Days

Reset days are not failed workout days. They are training days with a different assignment.

A reset day focuses on breath, posture, mobility, stability, walking, and light movement. It gives your body better signals without heavy stress.

Reset days are especially useful when you feel:

stiff

guarded

tired

tense

uneven

low energy

not ready for heavier loading

mentally drained but still needing movement

A reset day may include:

breathing work

Daily Structure Reset

Mobility Reset

light stability circuit

walking

gentle pattern practice

This kind of day protects consistency. It keeps you from falling into the all-or-nothing trap.

Many adults over 40 lose rhythm because they think every session must be intense to count. That is not true.

A reset day counts because it keeps the body connected. It keeps the habit alive. It keeps the structure moving. It gives the system a chance to recover while still receiving useful input.

Sometimes the smartest training day is the one that prevents the next setback.

Recovery Days

Recovery days are for restoration. That does not always mean lying on the couch all day. Sometimes full rest is needed. But often, recovery includes gentle movement, walking, hydration, sleep focus, nutrition, and lowering stress where possible.

A recovery day may include:

easy walking

light stretching if it feels good

breathing

hydration

better meals

earlier bedtime

no heavy training

no pressure to perform

Recovery days help the body adapt. They are where the work you already did has room to become progress.

If you never recover, the body never catches up. If you recover too much and never build, the body never gets challenged. The rhythm needs both.

Recovery is not quitting. It is how you keep building.

The Weekly Structure-First Template

A simple week does not need to be complex. Here is a basic structure-first rhythm:

Day 1 — Build

Day 2 — Reset or walk

Day 3 — Build

Day 4 — Recovery or light reset

Day 5 — Build

Day 6 — Reset, walk, or optional light strength

Day 7 — Recovery

This is only a template. It is not a command. Some people will do better with two build days per week. Some can handle three. Some may eventually handle four. Some need more reset days at first. Some need more walking. Some need shorter sessions. Some need more recovery because life stress is high.

The point is not to copy the template perfectly. The point is to understand the rhythm.

Build. Reset. Recover. Repeat.

If You Are Starting From Scratch

If you have been inactive, inconsistent, or uncertain, start smaller. A simple beginner week may look like this:

Day 1 — Build light

Day 2 — Walk + reset

Day 3 — Recovery

Day 4 — Build light

Day 5 — Walk + reset

Day 6 — Optional mobility or easy walk

Day 7 — Recovery

This is enough to start. Two build days can create progress if they are consistent. Two or three reset or walking days can restore rhythm. Recovery days help the body adapt.

The first goal is not to crush yourself. The first goal is to become the person who can repeat the week. Once you can repeat it, you can build it.

If You Already Train

If you already train consistently, the goal may not be to do more. It may be to organize better.

A trained person over 40 may need:

better warm-ups

better exercise selection

more deliberate mobility work

more stability before heavier loading

more recovery between intense sessions

fewer junk sets

better progression rules

more respect for readiness

A stronger weekly rhythm may look like this:

Day 1 — Build: lower-body emphasis

Day 2 — Reset + walk

Day 3 — Build: upper-body emphasis

Day 4 — Recovery or mobility

Day 5 — Build: full-body strength

Day 6 — Optional reset, walk, or light conditioning

Day 7 — Recovery

This keeps strength in the week. But it also protects the body from stacking intensity blindly. You still train hard. You just stop training randomly.

If Life Is Stressful

Some weeks are heavier than others. Work gets demanding. Sleep gets disrupted. Family needs increase. Travel happens. Stress rises. Schedules break.

This is where most people lose the rhythm. They either try to force the original plan or abandon it completely.

A structure-first week gives you a third option. Adjust.

If life stress is high, reduce training stress. That may mean:

fewer sets

lighter loads

shorter sessions

more reset work

more walking

more recovery

no training to failure

less aggressive progression

This is not weakness. It is load management. Stress counts as load. If life is already loading the system, training should be placed wisely.

You can still show up. But showing up may look different that week. That is how you preserve the long game.

The Low-Energy Week

There will be weeks when your body does not feel ready for normal training. Maybe sleep was poor. Maybe stress was high. Maybe you are stiff. Maybe your recovery is behind. Maybe your motivation is low.

Do not turn that week into failure. Use a low-energy week.

A low-energy week may look like this:

Day 1 — Daily Structure Reset + walk

Day 2 — Light mobility

Day 3 — Light strength circuit

Day 4 — Recovery

Day 5 — Daily Structure Reset + walk

Day 6 — Optional light movement

Day 7 — Recovery

The purpose is not to chase progress aggressively. The purpose is to keep rhythm. You maintain the habit. You keep the body moving. You reduce the chance of a full stop.

You protect the identity of someone who still cares for their body even when energy is low.

That matters. Because consistency is not built only on strong weeks. It is built by knowing what to do on weak weeks.

The Busy Week Minimum

Busy weeks are real. You may not have time for full workouts. But you can still keep the system alive.

A busy week minimum may be:

two short build sessions

two daily resets

two walks

one recovery day

That is enough to maintain momentum. A short build session might be twenty minutes. A reset might be five minutes. A walk might be ten to twenty minutes.

Do not underestimate small anchors. The body responds to repetition. The mind responds to kept promises.

When you keep the rhythm alive during a busy week, you avoid the emotional cost of starting over. You are not trying to do everything. You are protecting the chain.

The Weekly Readiness Review

At the end of each week, ask five questions:

Did I build?

Did I reset?

Did I recover?

What felt better?

What kept showing up?

This review should take less than five minutes. It keeps you from training blindly.

If your low back kept taking over, the next week may need more core-stack work. If your knees felt irritated, the next week may need more base control and less aggressive lower-body loading. If your shoulders felt better after reset work, keep that signal in the plan. If energy was low all week, recovery may need more attention. If strength improved and the body felt good, you may be ready to progress.

The weekly review helps you make better decisions. Not emotional decisions. Not guilt-based decisions. Structure-based decisions.

Progress the Week Slowly

Once a rhythm feels repeatable, you can progress it. But progress the week slowly.

Do not jump from two build days to five. Do not add weight, sets, exercises, and conditioning all at once. Do not turn a good week into an excuse to overload the next one.

Progress can come through:

adding one set

adding a small amount of load

adding one extra build day

adding a longer walk

improving range

improving control

increasing consistency

reducing pain or compensation

recovering faster

The weekly rhythm should grow like a structure. Layer by layer. Not randomly.

If you add too much too quickly, the body may push back. If you progress wisely, the body gains confidence.

The goal is not a perfect week. The goal is a repeatable week that can improve.

What To Do When You Miss Days

You will miss days. That is normal. Life will interrupt.

The mistake is turning a missed day into a missed week. Or a missed week into a lost month.

Do not punish yourself. Do not try to make up every missed workout by overloading the next session. That usually creates more problems.

Return to the rhythm. If you miss a build day, do the next planned session or use a lighter version. If you miss a reset day, do five minutes today. If you miss a full week, start with a low-energy week and rebuild.

The body does not need you to panic. It needs you to return.

Consistency is not never missing. Consistency is knowing how to come back.

WHAT THIS EXPLAINS

If you train hard for a few weeks and then fall off, your plan may be too intense to repeat.

If you keep getting stiff between workouts, your week may need more reset work.

If you feel beat up by the weekend, your build days may be too close together or too aggressive.

If you cannot stay consistent, you may need a minimum version for busy or low-energy weeks.

If your body improves when you walk more, walking may need to become part of the rhythm.

If your motivation rises when the week feels manageable, your system may finally match your life.

A good weekly rhythm does not only train the body. It protects momentum.

The Rhythm Becomes the Build

The goal is not to win one week. The goal is to build a rhythm that can carry you through many weeks.

That is how change happens. Not through one perfect plan. Through repeated structure.

You build. You reset. You recover. You review. You adjust. You repeat.

That is how your body learns. That is how strength becomes sustainable. That is how mobility becomes useful. That is how recovery becomes part of the system. That is how confidence returns.

A body after 40 does not need chaos. It needs cadence.

The next chapter will bring everything together into a simple starting plan. Not a forever plan. Not a perfect plan.

A first structure.

A four-week reset that helps you stop guessing and begin building with direction.

CHAPTER 14

The 4-Week Structure-First Reset Plan

Before you begin: Week 1 will feel slower than you expect. That is correct. The purpose of Week 1 is calibration, not training. You are learning your pattern, not fixing it. The fixing happens in Weeks 2 and 3. What you observe in Week 1 determines how useful everything after it actually is.

You do not need a perfect plan to begin. You need a clear first structure.

That is what this chapter gives you. Not a forever program. Not a medical protocol. Not an advanced training system. A starting plan.

A four-week reset designed to help you stop guessing, rebuild awareness, restore better movement, and begin training from a more organized foundation.

By this point, you have learned the major pieces:

Structure governs strength.

The body compensates.

The upper chain matters.

The core stack matters.

The base matters.

Assessment comes before intensity.

Recovery is part of training.

The week needs rhythm.

Now those ideas need to become action. Because understanding matters. But understanding must eventually become practice.

This plan is designed around one simple goal:

Help your body rebuild trust through structure.

Not by forcing. Not by rushing. Not by chasing soreness. By giving your body better signals for four straight weeks.

What This Plan Is Designed To Do

This plan is not designed to crush you. It is designed to organize you.

It helps you practice:

daily structure awareness

breathing and rib-pelvis control

upper-chain movement

hip and base awareness

mobility that transfers

stability before intensity

beginner strength patterns

recovery rhythm

weekly review

This plan is not trying to solve every issue. It is trying to give you a better starting point.

That matters. Because many adults over 40 do not fail because they need a more complicated program. They fail because they never build a repeatable foundation. They start too hard. They do too much. They skip assessment. They ignore recovery. They chase random exercises. Then when the body pushes back, they blame age, motivation, or discipline.

This plan gives you a different path.

Assess. Reset. Move. Build. Recover. Repeat.

Before You Start

Before beginning any exercise plan, use wisdom.

If you have sharp pain, numbness, tingling, swelling, sudden weakness, chest pain, dizziness, recent trauma, unexplained symptoms, or pain that does not settle, seek qualified guidance before pushing forward.

This plan is educational. It is not diagnosis. It is not treatment. It is a structure-first starting point.

This plan is a general starting structure. Adjust it to your body, your readiness, your equipment, and any guidance you have received from qualified professionals.

Move within a range you can control. Use support when needed. Modify anything that does not feel right. Stop anything that creates symptoms that concern you.

The goal is not to prove toughness. The goal is to rebuild trust.

The Four-Week Flow

The plan moves in phases. Each week has a different focus:

Week 1 — Awareness: Learn your patterns

Week 2 — Mobility + Control: Restore access

Week 3 — Foundation Strength: Build capacity

Week 4 — Integration: Train with confidence

This order matters. Most people want to jump straight to Week 3. They want the strength work. They want the results. They want to feel productive.

But after 40, the first two weeks are not wasted. They are preparation.

Week 1 teaches you what your body is showing you. Week 2 helps your body regain better options. Week 3 builds strength on top of better organization. Week 4 teaches you how to put the pieces together.

That is the structure-first path.

Week 1 — Awareness

The goal of Week 1 is to stop guessing.

This week is not about intensity. It is about learning. You are observing how your body stands, moves, breathes, balances, and responds. You are not trying to fix everything. You are gathering information.

Where do you feel stiff? Where do you feel unstable? Where does one side feel different? Where does the low back take over? Where does the neck tighten? Where do your knees shift? Where do your feet lose pressure? Where does your body feel better after a reset?

This week teaches you how to listen.

Week 1 Daily Practice

Each day, complete the Daily Structure Reset. This should take about five minutes.

Breathing Reset

Wall Posture Check

Upper-Back Opener

Hip Mobility Reset

Standing Stack Check

Move slowly. Do not force range. Do not rush. Your goal is to notice. Not perform.

After the reset, ask:

Do I feel more upright?

Do I feel more grounded?

Did one side feel different?

Did my neck, back, hips, or feet change?

Did any movement feel restricted?

Did anything feel better after a few minutes?

That information matters.

Week 1 Movement Days

Choose two or three days this week for light movement practice. This is not a full workout yet.

Squat-to-chair: 2 sets of 6–8

Hip hinge drill: 2 sets of 6–8

Wall push-up: 2 sets of 6–10

Light row or band pull if available: 2 sets of 8–10

Easy walk: 10–20 minutes

Keep the effort low to moderate. You should finish feeling better organized, not drained. If you do not have bands or weights, skip the row for now and focus on posture, walking, and the reset.

The goal is not to train hard. The goal is to see how your body responds to basic patterns.

Week 1 Reflection

At the end of the week, answer five questions:

What felt stiff most often?

What felt unstable?

What movement felt better after the reset?

What movement felt worse or more restricted?

What pattern kept showing up?

Do not judge the answers. Use them. This is your starting map.

Week 2 — Mobility + Control

The goal of Week 2 is to restore access.

Now that you have observed your patterns, you begin giving the body more movement options. Not extreme mobility. Usable mobility. The kind that helps you stand taller, reach better, hinge cleaner, squat with more control, walk with more confidence, and train without as much compensation.

This week continues the Daily Structure Reset, then adds the Mobility Reset.

Week 2 Daily Practice

Each day, complete the Daily Structure Reset. Then on three or four days, add the 10-Minute Mobility Reset:

Upper-Back Rotation

Shoulder Reach With Rib Control

Hip Shift

Hip Hinge Reach

Ankle Rock

Controlled Sit-to-Stand

This should not feel aggressive. Use small ranges if needed. Use support if needed. The goal is controlled access. Not forcing.

Week 2 Movement Days

Choose two or three days this week for light strength-pattern practice:

Squat-to-chair: 2–3 sets of 6–8

Hip hinge drill: 2–3 sets of 6–8

Split-stance hold: 2 rounds of 15–20 seconds per side

Wall push-up or elevated push-up: 2 sets of 6–10

Light row or band pull: 2 sets of 8–10

Easy walk: 10–25 minutes

Move slowly. Control the lowering. Breathe. Stop before form falls apart.

This is still not about heavy training. It is about teaching your body to access and control better positions.

Week 2 Reflection

At the end of the week, answer:

Which mobility movement felt most useful?

Which side felt more limited?

Did your walking, posture, or training feel different?

Did any tightness return less often?

What still feels guarded?

This helps you see what your body responds to. That response guides the next step.

Week 3 — Foundation Strength

The goal of Week 3 is to begin building capacity.

Now you will keep the reset work, but strength becomes more central. This is where many people want to overdo it. Do not rush.

The goal is not to prove strength. The goal is to build strength from structure. That means choosing versions of exercises your body can control. Not the hardest version. The right version.

Week 3 Weekly Rhythm

Day 1 — Build

Day 2 — Reset + walk

Day 3 — Build

Day 4 — Recovery or light reset

Day 5 — Build or light build

Day 6 — Walk + mobility

Day 7 — Recovery

If three build days feel like too much, use two. That is acceptable. Two good build days repeated consistently are better than three forced days that leave you beat up.

Week 3 Build Day Template

Start each build day with:

Quick Readiness Check

Daily Structure Reset

Mobility or Stability Prep

Strength Patterns

Recovery Finish

Then choose versions of these patterns you can control:

Squat pattern: 2–3 sets of 6–10

Hinge pattern: 2–3 sets of 6–10

Push pattern: 2–3 sets of 6–10

Pull pattern: 2–3 sets of 8–12

Carry or balance pattern: 2–3 rounds

Use light to moderate resistance. If you have no equipment, use bodyweight, a backpack, bands, or controlled tempo. The load should feel challenging, but not sloppy. Leave one to three good reps in reserve.

Week 3 Exercise Examples

Squat Pattern Options:

Squat-to-chair

Goblet squat to chair

Assisted squat

Box squat

Hinge Pattern Options:

Hip hinge drill

Dumbbell Romanian deadlift

Backpack hinge

Wall hinge

Push Pattern Options:

Wall push-up

Elevated push-up

Dumbbell press

Machine press

Pull Pattern Options:

Band row

Dumbbell row

Cable row

Machine row

Carry / Stability Options:

Suitcase carry

Farmer's carry

Split-stance hold

Controlled step-back

Choose the version your body can own. If the low back, neck, knees, or shoulders take over, adjust the exercise. That is not failure. That is assessment.

Week 3 Reflection

At the end of the week, answer:

Which strength pattern felt best?

Which pattern felt least controlled?

Did any exercise go to the wrong area?

Did recovery feel manageable?

What needs to be modified next week?

This is how the plan stays intelligent. The review keeps you from repeating the wrong pattern just because it was written down.

Week 4 — Integration

The goal of Week 4 is to bring the system together.

Assessment. Reset. Mobility. Stability. Strength. Recovery. Now you begin practicing the rhythm as a complete structure.

This week should help you feel more confident about what your body needs and how to train with less guessing. It is not the finish line. It is the first full cycle.

Week 4 Weekly Rhythm

Day 1 — Build

Day 2 — Reset + walk

Day 3 — Build

Day 4 — Recovery

Day 5 — Build

Day 6 — Mobility + walk

Day 7 — Recovery + review

Adjust if needed. If your body is not recovering well, reduce one build day. If your body feels strong and controlled, progress slightly. The goal is to learn the rhythm.

Week 4 Build Day Template

Each build day follows the same order: Assess. Reset. Prepare. Build. Recover.

A simple build session may look like this:

Daily Structure Reset: 5 minutes

Mobility or stability prep: 5–10 minutes

Squat pattern: 3 sets of 6–10

Push or pull pattern: 3 sets of 8–12

Hinge or carry pattern: 2–3 sets

Easy walk or breathing finish: 5 minutes

Keep the work clean. Do not chase exhaustion. Chase repeatable quality. A good session should challenge you and still leave you able to come back.

How To Progress During Week 4

Progress gently. Choose only one progression at a time. You can:

add one set

add two reps

slow the lowering

increase range slightly

reduce support

add light resistance

add a short carry

improve control

improve consistency

Do not add everything at once. The body needs clear signals. If you change too many variables, you will not know what helped or what irritated the pattern.

Progress should feel earned. Not forced.

What If Week 4 Still Feels Hard?

That is okay. The goal of four weeks is not perfection. It is direction.

If Week 4 still feels hard, repeat the plan. Or repeat Week 2 or Week 3. There is no shame in repeating a phase. Repetition is how the body learns.

If mobility still feels limited, spend more time in Week 2. If strength feels unstable, repeat Week 3. If recovery feels poor, adjust the rhythm. If pain or symptoms concern you, seek qualified guidance.

The plan is not a prison. It is a map. Use it. Adjust it. Build from it.

What You Should Notice After Four Weeks

Everyone responds differently. But after four weeks of structure-first work, you may notice:

better awareness of your posture

less guessing before workouts

improved breathing awareness

better control in basic movements

more confidence with squats, hinges, pushes, pulls, or carries

better understanding of what tightness means

clearer signs of when to train, reset, or recover

less fear around movement

stronger weekly rhythm

better consistency

You may not feel completely different. That is not the only measure. The first win is clarity. You are learning your body again. You are building a foundation. You are moving from random effort to structured practice.

That is progress.

WHAT THIS EXPLAINS

If you have struggled with consistency, you may not have needed more motivation. You may have needed a plan that gave you options for different kinds of days.

If workouts kept leaving you beat up, you may have needed a better entry point before adding intensity.

If stretching alone never changed much, you may have needed mobility with control.

If strength work always went to the wrong areas, you may have needed assessment and stability first.

If you kept starting over, you may have needed a rhythm that could survive real life.

The four-week reset helps you stop treating every workout like a separate event. It teaches you to see training as a system.

The Plan Is the Beginning

At the end of four weeks, you are not finished. You are clearer. That is the point.

You should have a better sense of:

what your body responds to

what patterns need attention

what exercises feel useful

what areas compensate

what kind of weekly rhythm you can repeat

what level of strength work your body can tolerate

what recovery demands respect

Before you jump to the next thing, review what the plan showed you. Your body gave you information. Use it.

If your upper chain still feels restricted, keep working the upper-chain reset. If your core stack still feels disorganized, keep building breathing, bracing, and trunk control. If your base still feels unstable, keep working foot pressure, hip control, balance, and strength patterns.

If strength feels ready, progress gradually. If recovery is still inconsistent, fix the rhythm before chasing harder work.

The next step should come from the map. Not from panic. Not from boredom. Not from comparison. From clarity.

From Reset to Build

The four-week reset is designed to get you started. But eventually, the goal is to build.

Build strength. Build mobility. Build stability. Build capacity. Build confidence. Build a body you trust.

The reset gives you the foundation. The build continues the process.

That is why this book does not end with a perfect plan. It gives you a way to think. A way to listen. A way to train. A way to adjust. A way to keep moving forward.

Your body is not asking for random effort. It is asking for direction.

And now you have a starting structure.

The next step is learning how to use what this plan revealed.

Because the goal is not only to complete four weeks.

The goal is to understand what your body has been explaining all along.

CHAPTER 15

What This Explains

By now you have a framework for reading your body differently. When the shoulder tightens on a press, you ask what the ribcage is doing. When the low back grabs during a hinge, you ask whether the hips are actually folding or just borrowing from the lumbar. When the neck tightens on a carry, you ask whether the shoulder blades are doing their job or whether the traps are covering for them.

That shift — from chasing symptoms to reading patterns — is what this book was designed to produce. Structure governs strength. Assessment comes before intensity. Reset before you load. The body tells you what it needs if you know how to listen.

The four-week plan gave you a starting point. What you noticed during it gave you a direction. Use both. The plan is a map. The body is the territory. Keep reading the territory.

> *The patterns that showed up are not permanent. They are current. And current patterns can be changed with better inputs, consistently applied.*

CHAPTER 16

From General Map to Personal Assessment

A book can give you the map. But your body still has its own pattern. That distinction matters.

Everything in this book has given you language. You understand that stiffness can be a signal. Weakness can be a signal. Compensation deserves respect rather than force. Structure governs what strength can do. Assessment comes before intensity. Reset work gives the body better signals before loading asks it to produce.

That language is useful. But a general map cannot tell you whether your right hip drives differently than your left, whether your shoulder blade control is the limiting factor in your press, or whether your upper-back rotation is actually improving or just getting borrowed from the lower back.

If you can continue on your own, begin with the four-week reset. Use what you observed. Build from there. If certain patterns keep returning despite consistent work, or if you are unsure which area to prioritize, a structure-first assessment can give you the clarity a general program cannot.

Your body is not broken. It has a pattern. And once that pattern is seen clearly, it can be rebuilt with better structure.

> *The book gives the map. The assessment gives the mirror. The program gives the build.*

www.ingramcontent.com/pod-product-compliance
Lightning Source LLC
LaVergne TN
LVHW010658110826
845149LV00014B/3146
* 9 7 9 8 9 9 6 2 4 5 5 2 9 *